MW00903483

INNOVATION
and
PERSEVERANCE

A History of the Tulane University
Department of Surgery

Matthew D. Zelhart, MD
Douglas P. Slakey, MD

Copyright © 2013 Matthew D. Zelhart, MD and Douglas P. Slakey, MD
ISBN: 1490366458
ISBN 13: 9781490366456

Dedication

To the surgeons of New Orleans who are devoted
to training the next generation.

Preface

When Hurricane Katrina struck New Orleans in 2005, it not only disrupted the lives of the residents of New Orleans, but also destroyed many of the historical records in the city. Charity Hospital, for example, kept their medical records in the basement of the hospital. After the flood, these records were lost, greatly complicating future patient care. The flooding at Tulane University School of Medicine resulted in a loss of documentation and artifacts as well. When the medical school reopened, there was not even a record of the past chairs of the Department of Surgery, a travesty for a department with such a distinguished history.

The destruction of Katrina created an impetus for us to consolidate the history of the Department of Surgery into one book. Years of work have been put into compiling this story, starting with the work of Christopher Harter of the Amistad Foundation a few years after Katrina. Further detail has been obtained from Rudolph Matas's *History of Medicine in New Orleans*, John Duffy's *History of Tulane University Medical Center*, and historical documents. Further, many interviews have been conducted to fill in the gaps and to record the modern history of the department.

The book is written in two parts. Because Hurricane Katrina was such a significant and devastating event that led to the creation of this book, we have given it a section alone. The first section describes firsthand accounts of Hurricane Katrina and the rebuilding process afterward. The second part is a more traditional chronological record of the department. As you will see, the history of the department is quite an illustrious story.

Part I

Hurricane Katrina formed over the Bahamas on August 23, 2005. It continued to gain power over the warm waters of the Gulf of Mexico, quickly becoming a category 3 storm. Preparing for disaster, the City of New Orleans issued the first mandatory evacuation order in its history on August 28. Katrina finally made landfall in Southeast Louisiana on August 29.

As the storm grew over the Gulf of Mexico, so did the concerns about the damage and destruction it would bring. Tulane University Medical Center began making emergency plans in preparation for the impending disaster. As many noncritical patients as possible were immediately discharged or evacuated from the hospital. However, there were many critical patients who were not stable enough for an immediate evacuation. As this reality set in, the hospital began making preparations to wait out the impending storm.

On Sunday the 28, hurricane on-call and volunteer staff were encouraged to go home and grab clothes, food, and supplies. They were unsure how long the hospital would be isolated from the rest of the world, and they were encouraged to prepare for the worst. When the mandatory evacuation was declared, the decision was made that families and pets of the emergency staff would be able to wait out the storm at the hospital along with their working family members. Throughout Sunday afternoon and evening, families and pets filed into the hospital—a modern day Noah's Ark. The surgery residents, staff, and nurses occupied rooms in the same-day surgical center, filling them with their belongings and sleeping on the patient stretchers already in the rooms.[1]

At the same time, many people began taking shelter at the nearby Superdome, which was to be a "shelter of last resort."[2] As the numbers in the Superdome began to swell to over twenty-five thousand people, it became clear that they were not well equipped to handle the many people with chronic medical conditions. Officials then arranged for the transfer of people with critical medical conditions to Tulane University, mainly those with dialysis-dependent end-stage renal disease, severe diabetes, and in-home medical needs. In all, sixty patients and their families were transferred to the Tulane Medical Center and were housed in the Post-Anesthesia Care Unit (PACU). Their care would be managed by the surgical teams that remained in the hospital.[3]

By Sunday evening, the hospital was locked down, and the occupants went to bed as the rain began to fall. The storm reached its peak around one on Monday morning. The howling wind whistled through the hospital, and water leaked in through weak areas of the structure, but all in all the facility seemed to be weathering the storm well. Around three in the morning, the hospital lost power, but the generators quickly kicked in—as was the norm for many previous New Orleans hurricanes. The next morning, the hospital began to awaken and resume post-hurricane activities without much excitement. Many had breakfast in the first-floor cafeteria and looked outside to survey the damage and the surrounding area. Around ten on Monday morning, it seemed to be the beginning of a beautiful day outside. The Crescent City was picturesque—

---

1   Interview with Ron Stein, November 15, 2012.
2   Lise Olsen, "City Had Evacuation Plan but Strayed from Strategy," *Houston Chronicle*, September 8, 2005.
3   Interview with Ron Stein, November 15, 2012.

clear and sunny. Downed branches and power lines littered the street, but for the most part, the city appeared dry. At this point, many felt that the storm had been overhyped and that the relief team would be in later that day. The residents and staff even had a toga party, using bed sheets and hallway plants for costumes, to pass the time. This feeling, however, would not last much longer.[4]

Throughout the rest of the morning and the early part of the afternoon, many people noticed more water in the street. This seemed peculiar since the hospital is not in a part of the city that gets a lot of flooding, but the oddity was brushed aside at first, and many thought nothing of it.[5]

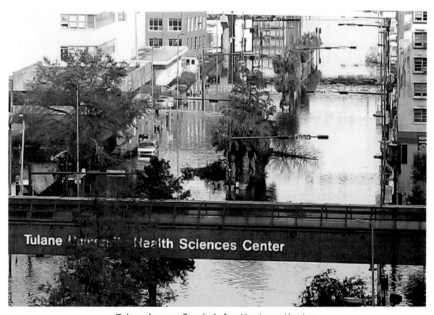

Tulane Avenue flooded after Hurricane Katrina.

In the early evening on Monday, word got to the hospital that the levees had broken. Those who had long lived in New

---

4   Interview with Bernard Jaffe, November 14, 2012.
5   Interview with Norman McSwain, November 16, 2012.

Orleans knew what this meant, and for a few, panic began to set in. There had been reports for years of a "doomsday" for New Orleans if the levees built by the Army Corps of Engineers ever broke; however, funding for strengthening the levees always seemed to be funneled to more urgent and demanding issues. Little concern was given to the levees, which had been around for decades. As night fell on Monday, August 29, many went to bed uneasy and unsure of when help would arrive.

The storm surge caused more than fifty breaches in drainage canals and navigational canal levees and precipitated the worst engineering disaster in the history of the United States. By August 31, 2005, 80 percent of New Orleans was flooded, with some parts under fifteen feet of water.[6] Some areas of the city would stay that way for weeks.

When people awoke Tuesday morning, they found that water had risen substantially. Residents quickly moved the Tulane University supplies and personnel to higher ground. They then transferred as much food as possible from the first-floor cafeteria to be distributed among staff and patients. The residents carried the pharmacy supplies to the endoscopy center and moved central supply into the actual operating rooms— all on the third floor of the hospital. The nurses unlocked and immediately removed all drugs from the electronic pixus machines, which normally hold the hospital's medications. The hospital was now on lockdown, and security began carrying automatic weapons.[7]

---

6   Dan Swenson, "Flash Flood: Hurricane Katrina's Inundation of New Orleans," *Time-Picayune*, August 29, 2005.
7   Interview with Ron Stein, November 15, 2012.

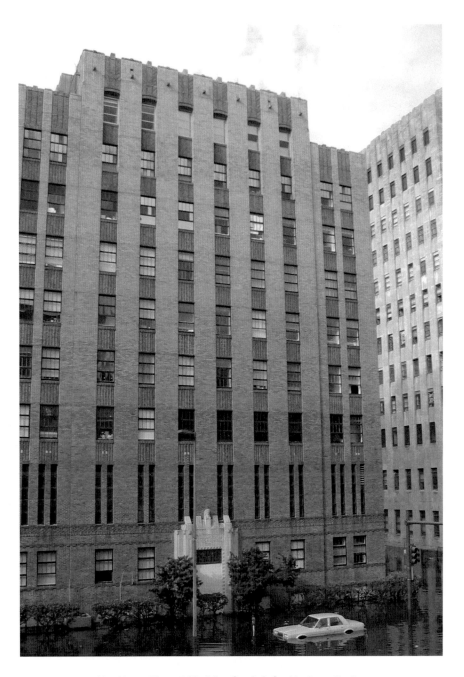

Hutchinson Memorial Building flooded after Hurricane Katrina.

As the water rose, the hospital infrastructure was breached early Tuesday morning. The backup generators were housed on the ground floor, and the water seeping in flooded the generators, causing backup power to fail. Near this time, water pressure in the hospital was lost as well. By noon on Tuesday, six to eight feet flooded the hospital, which now had no power and no fresh water. When one peered outside, the topography was completely changed, and all you could see in the streets was water. Where there were once mailboxes, downed tree limbs, and street signs, now only a vast sheet of water existed.[8]

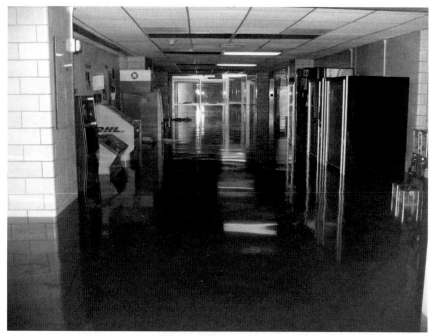

First floor of the Tulane School of Medicine flooded after Hurricane Katrina.

After the storm, the landscape of the city was littered with people stranded on their roofs after they had cut their way through their attics, often using hatchets, to escape the rising floodwaters. There were many floating bodies of those who

---

8   Interview with Bernard Jaffe, November 14, 2012.

were not so lucky. Streets became a grid of rivers, and rescue boats with volunteers went out on missions throughout the city.

Those staying in the hospital quickly realized that help would not come soon. They were stranded in a desolate hospital island with critical ICU patients. Since all power was out, patients who were intubated would now have to be bag-ventilated by hand. Many family members of patients and of the staff volunteered around the clock to keep these people alive. The dialysis-dependent patients were no longer able to get the lifeline they needed to replace their kidneys. In fact, several dialysis-dependent patients sent over from the Superdome went into comas before they were ultimately evacuated. The hospital staff cared for patients in complete darkness, sloshing through the water that had leaked in through the storm and over the past day.[9]

It was at this point that some who remained in the city began to panic. By August 30, looting for essential survival goods was rampant throughout the city. Gangs of roaming gunmen went through the city, unchecked by an exhausted police force. On Tuesday, many of the occupants at Tulane Medical Center looked out the window and saw massive looting of the Walgreens and drug stores adjacent to the hospital. Images of mothers carrying diapers over their heads and families trying to secure fresh water from convenience stores will not soon be forgotten.

Throughout the chaos, rumors of martial law began to sweep though the city. Conditions had forced staff to move patients from their rooms to more secure areas away from windows. As the temperature rose in the city, conditions became worse in the hospital. With no air conditioning and windows that did not open, the building turned into a sauna, with the sun beating down on an already humid city covered in water. Many staff took scissors to their scrubs, turning them into shorts and tank tops; they also used pulse-e-vacs in an attempt

---

9   Interview with Bernard Jaffe, November 14, 2012.

to keep cool. Many patients had temperatures rising to 104°F, forcing medical staff to douse them with alcohol, having no other options to battle fever.[10]

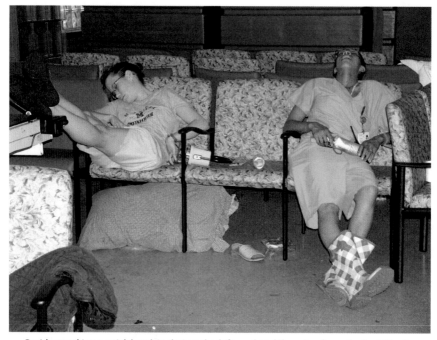

Residents taking a quick break in their makeshift scrubs while caring for patients at Charity Hospital during Hurricane Katrina.

It became clear that evacuations of patients, staff, and other people would be absolutely necessary. The hospital managing company, Hospital Corporation of America (HCA), decided to begin helicopter evacuations from the hospital Tuesday night. At the time, it was not certain if the hospital infrastructure was strong enough to allow a helicopter to land on the roof. It was determined that the helicopters would have to land on the Saratoga parking structure attached to the hospital. Because

10 Interview with Bernard Jaffe, November 14, 2012.

curfews were being enforced at that time, evacuations could be carried out only during daylight hours.[11]

On Tuesday evening, evacuations began, starting with patients in the Pediatric ICU (PICU). Intubated children were brought down, being hand ventilated by their nurses. Since the evacuation helicopters were small, only the child and his or her nurse were allowed to be transported. Heartbreaking scenes took place on the roof of the parking facility—mothers and fathers had to say goodbye to their children, having no idea where their children would end up or if they would even survive the journey. The children were taken immediately to the airport to be rerouted, or else they would learn of the accepting facilities in route and thus adjust their course. The PICU nurses were the only lifeline many of the parents had to their very sick children.

The looting and "mayhem" taking place in the city were hampering efforts to evacuate the Tulane Medical Center. "If we do not have the federal presence in New Orleans tonight at dark, it will no longer be safe to be there, hospital or no hospital," Acadian Ambulance Services CEO Richard Zuschlag told CNN on August 31 in regard to the evacuation of the medical district.[12]

On August 31, New Orleans's 1,500-member police force was ordered to abandon search-and-rescue missions and turn its attention toward controlling the widespread looting. The city also ordered a mandatory curfew. Mayor Nagin called for increased federal assistance in a "desperate S.O.S." following the city's inability to control looting.[13]

When evacuation efforts resumed the next day, they were met with a volley of gunfire. Armed men had broken into the dialysis center across from the parking garage and fired at helicopters trying to land and take off. SWAT teams arrived, and staff and patients took cover behind the walls of the crosswalk as authori-

11 Interview with Rodney Steiner, December 5, 2012.
12 "Mayhem Hampering Hospital Evacuations," *CNN*, August 31, 2005.
13 Justin Borger, "Mayor Issues SOS as Chaos Tightens Its Grip," *Guardian*, September 2, 2005.

ties got the situation under control. After multiple lost hours, the evacuation resumed with renewed urgency.[14]

On Wednesday, the critical patients were evacuated next. A team of nurses and doctors went through the hospital triaging patients so that the most critical patients could be evacuated first. Many end-stage renal disease patients had been without dialysis for days and were struggling. Army trucks and airboats transported ICU patients from Charity across the street to the Saratoga parking structure for evacuation. At the time, Tulane had a robust bariatric surgery program. Getting these patients out of the hospital and onto the roof of a parking garage with no working elevators posed many challenges. One six-hundred-pound patient had to be duct taped to a mattress and slid down a back stairwell from the seventh floor of the hospital to the second-floor crosswalk.[15] They then loaded the patient onto the back of a pickup truck and drove to the roof of the parking structure. Dr. Bernard Jaffe had done a bypass on a 550-pound eighteen-year-old woman in the days immediately before the storm. He and his team carried her from the third-floor ICU to the second-floor parking structure—going far beyond the normal postsurgical care. She was the last patient evacuated, leaving on Wednesday, August 31. After the patients were evacuated, their family members and the family members of the staff were evacuated by helicopter. Those with pets were taken by boat and driven to the airport.[16]

---

14 Interview with Ron Stein, November 15, 2012.
15 Interview with Ron Stein, November 15, 2012.
16 Interview with Ron Stein, November 15, 2012.

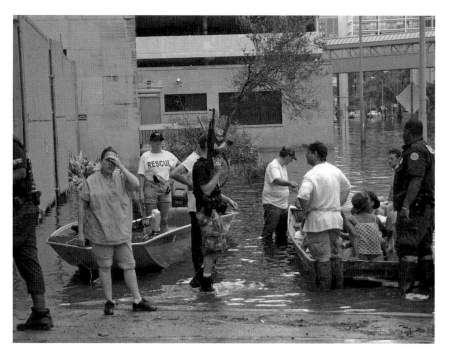

Hospital personnel taking patients from Charity Hospital to the Tulane parking garage to reach the helicopter.

By Thursday, September 1, the last staff members were evacuated from the hospital. Amazingly, despite all the mayhem, not a single patient died at Tulane Hospital. Helicopters took the exhausted staff to the airport, and their shoes and clothes were confiscated and incinerated for fear of contamination. By Friday, they had reached an HCA hospital in Lafayette, decontaminated, and started on prophylactic ciprofloxacin.

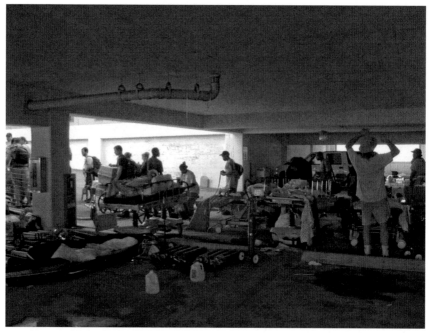

The last of the Tulane staff being evacuated by helicopter from the roof of the parking garage.

With all the tragedy surrounding Hurricane Katrina, there were also amazing stories of survival. One story in particular involved a dog named Moose. Dr. Rodney Steiner had been a pediatric surgeon at Tulane since 1993 and had stayed at the hospital to take care of patients during the storm. Steiner's wife, his four children, and their 115-pound Labrador named Moose all stayed in his office to weather the storm. When word came that the only reliable way out would be via helicopter, the family realized they would have to leave the dog behind. Knowing that it was very unlikely they would ever see Moose again, with tears in their eyes, they secured as much fresh water and food as they could from the vivarium in the medical school. They then papered the floor and locked Moose in the copy room of the surgery department, abandoning him on Wednesday night. Word quickly spread that a dog had been left behind in the surgery department. A plastic surgery fellow heard the story and was able to reenter the city to check on her house a week later. She decided to rescue Moose while there if at all possible. She drove in her old Range Rover toward the hospital until the water was too deep, which was about half a mile away. There, she found a man with a motorboat that was unfortunately out of gas who agreed to row them to the hospital. At one point along their journey, the National Guard stopped them, but they explained their mission and even got a soldier to give up his flashlight! They rowed all the way to the medical school and broke in through a door in the parking garage. They reached the surgery department and started looking around—they finally located Moose when he started barking. They opened the door to the copy room, to an obvious mess, and coaxed Moose out and into the boat.[17] The next day she drove to Houston, with Moose's paws on the dashboard and his head out the sunroof the entire journey, to reunite Moose with the Steiner family.

Of the twenty-five thousand people who took shelter at the Superdome—which was meant to be a shelter of last resort—six deaths resulted: one suicide, one overdose, and four of natural causes.[18] It was not until September 4 that the entire Superdome was evacuated. The sixty patients and their families who were transferred to Tulane were all evacuated to safety and survived, even though some were comatose from lack of dialysis or uncontrolled blood sugars.

In all, 1,464 people lost their lives in the city of New Orleans as a result of Hurricane Katrina.

***

Like the city of New Orleans, the Department of Surgery was in shambles after the storm. Staff and residents were scat-

---

17 Interview with Rodney Steiner, December 5, 2012.
18 Brian Thevenot, "Reports of Anarchy at Superdome Overstated," *Seattle Times*, September 26, 2005.

tered throughout the country, and there was no predetermined or organized way of contacting everyone. All the records and phone numbers of the residents and staff were at the surgery department offices in a building that would not be accessible until February of 2006.

A week after the evacuation of Tulane, members of the Department of Surgery began contacting each other through the Tulane Transplant website, whose server was housed outside New Orleans. As the members of the department came together, it was clear that Tulane's downtown campus and Charity Hospital would not be open for some time. Staff began working at hospitals outside the city, each able to take only a few residents. At the same time, the entire 2005 intern class was moved to Houston, where it was determined that they would finish their residency.[19]

Within one month, Tulane Lakeside Hospital reopened. The hospital was previously the women's and children's hospital and had been acquired by Tulane shortly before the storm. Lakeside Hospital was one of the few hospitals open right after the storm in the city of New Orleans. Lakeside Hospital was staffed by Drs. James Korndorffer and Ralph Corsetti and two second-year residents. Dr. Steve Jones replaced Dr. Ralph Corsetti later in 2006 and was joined part time by Dr. James Brown.

Dr. James Korndorffer recounts eerie scenes of life in New Orleans and driving back and forth from his house in the city to Lakeside Hospital in the suburb of Metairie right after the storm: stopping through National Guard checkpoints both ways, sitting on his porch at night deafened by stark silence, and eating at the only diner open for months and never seeing a woman or child in the city. Immediately after the storm, only critical personnel were allowed in the city—most of these being National Guard or those working to rebuild the city's infrastructure. Jim Korndorffer still remembers the first time

---

19 Interview with Doug Slakey, November 15, 2012.

after the storm seeing a child in the city and being struck with how odd it was to see children in New Orleans again after such a long time.[20]

In stark contrast to the desolation at home, Lakeside Hospital was bustling. Being one of the few hospitals open, especially one with surgical capabilities, ensured a constant stream of patients. Patients constantly filled the operating rooms, with the general surgeons operating on approximately seven patients each per day, sometimes up to six days a week.[21]

In addition to Lakeside, the other Tulane staff quickly stepped into place around Southeast Louisiana to serve the needs of the community. Dr. Douglas Slakey immediately went to Lakeview Hospital on the other side of Lake Pontchartrain in Covington, Louisiana, to begin rebuilding the transplant program. He also had residents working with him at that site.[22]

After rescuers evacuated Dr. Jaffe from Tulane Hospital, he went to Boston. He was contacted and asked to return to Louisiana to the Earl K. Long Hospital in Pineville, Louisiana. After spending a little over a week recovering from Katrina, Dr. Jaffe began work at one of the Charity system's key hospitals, now that the Charity Hospital in New Orleans was nonfunctional. Dr. Jaffe led a busy practice there and even contacted and cared for the bariatric patient whom he had carried down the steps in the evacuation of Tulane. Dr. Jaffe had five residents working with him at Pineville.[23]

Dr. Norman McSwain worked to reopen a trauma facility in New Orleans. Immediately after the storm, he worked at the hospital in Elmwood, Louisiana. He and Dr. Mary Jo Wright worked side by side with Drs. John Hunt and Alan Marr from LSU. Together, they worked to open the Spirit of Charity Trauma Center in New Orleans. Dr. McSwain's collaborative work with LSU faculty led to the integration of the Tulane and

---

20 Interview with Jim Korndorffer, November 12, 2012.
21 Interview with Jim Korndorffer, November 12, 2012.
22 Interview with Doug Slakey, November 15, 2012.
23 Interview with Bernard Jaffe, November 14, 2012.

LSU trauma surgeons in the new combined trauma service at Charity, whereas previously the Tulane and LSU surgical services were completely separate entities. In the old Charity system, there were *T* and *L* days, where the only trauma service to care for new patients on *T* days was Tulane, and the only trauma service to care for new trauma patients on the *L* days was LSU. Now, both programs saw the need to combine and work together with their limited resources to create an efficient and cooperative integrated trauma team for the patients of New Orleans. This integration for trauma services still exists today and is currently the model for other services and subspecialties to work together efficiently in the Charity system.[24]

In addition to the residents in Houston, other residents spread out between Pineville, New Orleans, Metairie, and Covington. It was clear that this arrangement could not last, or else the residency program could not survive. At the time, rotations to different sites between the residents was not possible. For example, those at Pineville stayed at Pineville with no plans to leave or get relief. Those involved felt confusion and uncertainty about the best course for the future of the department. Dr. Hewitt, who was chair of the department, had not yet returned from the evacuation, and it was unclear when he would. Tulane's downtown campus was months from opening, and no one was able to access any of the records.[25]

With the reformation of the program at a standstill, the working members of the Department of Surgery decided that they would meet with the residents and determine the future of the program. The residents met with Drs. Slakey and Jaffe at Prejeans restaurant in Lafayette, Louisiana. This would turn out to be a pivotal moment for the future of the department. The program was in shambles and scattered around the state, even into Texas. All involved could have simply walked away and let the program close. However, it was clear to all at the

---

24 Interview with Norman McSwain, November 16, 2012.
25 Interview with Jim Korndorffer, November 12, 2012.

infamous meeting at Prejeans that the Tulane Department of Surgery was something special and something worth fighting for. With this, staff began to set up official rotations and contact the Residency Review Committee (RRC) to begin the process of continuing with the program for the next cycle.[26]

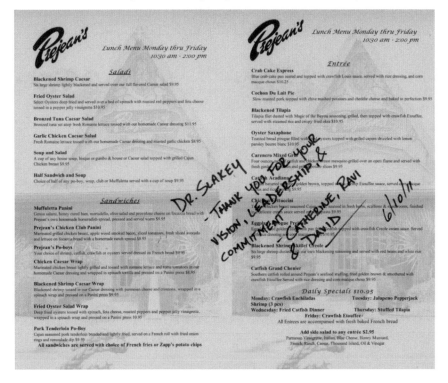

One of the signed Prejeans menus given to Drs. Korndorffer and Slakey by the residents to thank them for their dedication in reforming the program.

At this time, the Tulane School of Medicine building still had not reopened, and staff were still unable to access the old records. Dr. Korndorffer became acting director of the residency program, compiling the paperwork for submission to the RRC. The meetings at Prejeans continued, and residents rotated to different sites to help diversify their resident educa-

26 Interview with Doug Slakey, November 15, 2012.

tion. Even though Tulane Downtown had not reopened and the old administration was still not taking an active role, things seemed to be moving in the right direction.

As 2006 began, Dr. Hewitt's wife's battle with cancer became known. As he had still not returned to New Orleans, he stepped down as chair of the department in order to spend more time with his wife. In February 2006, everyone agreed that Dr. Slakey was the clear choice for the position of department chair. The RRC made a site visit within one month of Dr. Slakey taking the chair position. Their report, delivered months later, was a shock that would markedly change the course of the department.

Looking at the data from September to December 2005, the RRC felt that the population size in New Orleans did not warrant and could not sustain three residency programs (Tulane, Ochsner, and LSU). They mandated an "expedited withdrawal" of the Tulane surgery program, essentially a death sentence. In their correspondence, they noted, "The proposal for expedited withdrawal for accreditation is based on a catastrophic loss of resources, including faculty, facilities, and funding; and egregious noncompliance with accreditation requirements as listed: The operative experience available for resident education is insufficient and imbalanced. The proposed and current institutional sites do not support a quality education program…Resident supervision and the faculty-resident ratio are noncompliant."[27]

With this devastating condemnation, Drs. Slakey and Korndorffer suspended their responsibilities rebuilding the hospital and immediately dug through old records of the previous leadership in the Department of Surgery to ascertain the historic basis of the RRC's accusations. They rose to the difficult challenge, made more so by the fact the medical school build-

---

27 Doris Stoll, "Residency Review Committee Evaluation for Tulane University" (letter), December 5, 2006

ing was not fully open for access to these records until later in 2006.[28]

When the staff finally collected and reviewed the records, it became clear that the Tulane surgery residency before the storm, being one of the oldest programs in the country, was desperately trying to hold on to the old "Charity way" of conducting itself and was, therefore, not meeting current expectations of the Surgery RRC. It became apparent that university officials outside the previous department chair's office did not know the extent of the problems that the surgery residency program had before the storm. The program had received yearly citations from the RRC for "deficiencies in defined categories of cases" throughout the early 2000s. In fact, "even when minimum numbers were met, the breadth of cases was insufficient and in some case categories the numbers were below the 10th percentile level, which the Committee considers a grossly noncompliant experience." In addition, many of the residents operated with little, or completely without, attending supervision—which had been the norm for Charity training for the last century. Furthermore, the program had a dismal matriculation rate, and the entire fourth-year residency class was fired before the storm even came.[29]

Anxiety spread through the department and the School of Medicine, with many calling for a legal appeal of the decision. Unfortunately, in consideration of all that was discovered about how the program had operated prior to Katrina, Dr. Slakey and the remaining faculty agreed that the RRC's points were valid and true. In consultation with university president Scott Cowan and hospital leadership, they decided to voluntarily withdrawal the existing residency and immediately apply as a new, radically redesigned program, in hopes for a seamless transition to the next academic year. At this time, the department officially made Dr. Korndorffer the new program director.[30]

---

28 Interview with Doug Slakey, November 15, 2012.
29 Interview with Jim Korndorffer, November 12, 2012.
30 Interview with Jim Korndorffer, November 12, 2012.

To create the new structure of the general surgery department, Dr. Slakey met with multiple consultants, including the Yale surgery department, which had recently withdrawn their program and reformed as a new residency. It became clear that the operative experience at Tulane and the Spirit of Charity would no longer be enough. Traditionally, Tulane had not wanted residents to work outside of its institution, but Drs. Slakey and Korndorffer went out into the community and began forming relationships with the "nonacademic" surgeons of New Orleans. Since Katrina, talks had been in place with Dr. Jeff Griffin and the surgeons at East Jefferson Hospital to place residents in their practices. This initial relationship was a great success. As Slakey and Korndorffer went out through the community, they fostered relationships with surgeons at West Jefferson Hospital, Touro Infirmary, and Children's Hospital.[31] In addition, they recruited new faculty to join the Tulane Department of Surgery. The department added thirteen new full-time teaching faculty and fifteen clinical teaching faculty. Full-time teaching faculty included Drs. James Brown, Ernest Chiu, Juan Duchesne, Paul Friedlander, Steve Jones, Emad Kandil, Mary Killackey, Clifton McGinness, Jennifer McGee, Peter Meade, Anil Paramesh, Mary Jo Wright, and Thomas Yeh. The clinical faculty included Drs. Brent Alper, Todd Belott, Gustavo Colon, Jay Gillmore, Jeff Griffin, Richard Karlin, Gene Kukuy, Emery Minnard, Sean Mayfield, Nick Moustoukas, Robert Normand, Nalini Raju, David Treen, Robert Uddo, and Rubin Zhang.[32]

Furthermore, the department placed an emphasis on education and recruited Peggy Chehardy, EdD, as the director of the division of surgical education. She worked to create an educational curriculum for the residents. Drs. Slakey and Korndorffer developed goals and objectives for every surgical rotation. Along with Dr. Edward Newsome, who became chief of plastic surgery in late 2005, they completely redesigned the

---

31 Interview with Doug Slakey, November 15, 2012.
32 Jim Korndorffer, "Program Information Form" (letter).

residency program. Morbidity and mortality conferences and grand rounds had been poorly attended before the storm. Now they were a weekly occurrence, along with additional resident education conferences, such as basic surgical science curriculums. ABSITE scores, which would sometimes average in the single digits before the storm, quickly rose.[33]

After the storm, the plastic surgery department was also in disarray. Dr. Edward Newsome led the reformation. Dr. Newsome had joined the Tulane plastic surgery department after finishing his training in 1998. He was known for his passionate work on skin cancers, limb disfigurements, and reconstruction. After the storm, he worked tirelessly to bring the plastic surgery fellowship program back to Tulane and to form joint conferences with the LSU department. Tragically, in 2009, an unknown intruder murdered Dr. Newsome in his French Quarter home, which was subsequently burned with his body inside. The case remains unsolved to this day.[34]

The department sent the new, modernized surgical program proposal to the RRC in early 2007. The department then had to wait for word on whether or not it would be approved. The RRC did not allow the department to participate in the match during that time, so it was not allowed to actively recruit an incoming intern class to begin in July 2007, even if it was accredited. To remedy this, after the match, they offered three Tulane medical students intern positions contingent upon the program becoming accredited. They promised these three optimistic Tulane students a paid research year and help in finding a residency in the event that the new Tulane surgery residency application was not approved, a tremendous leap of faith for both parties. On June 28, days before the July 1 start date, the RRC accredited the program for three residency positions each year and a two-year accreditation cycle—the

---

33 Stoll, "Residency Review Committee."
34 Charles Dupin, "Memoir," http://www.aaps1921.org/memoirs/edwardnewsome.cgi (accessed February 1, 2013).

maximum allowed for a new program.[35] Two years later, they reaccredited the program for the maximum five years, and the complement of residents increased to four each year. Tulane is now one of the most modern surgery programs, redesigned out of necessity and the aftermath of Katrina, with a history as being the third-oldest program in the country. Tulane's residency program continues to thrive, receiving nearly one thousand applications for the four categorical positions in 2012.[36]

---

35 Interview with Jim Korndorffer, November 12, 2012.
36 Interview with Jim Korndorffer, November 12, 2012.

Part II

History of Tulane University Department of Surgery

The mission of the Tulane University Department of Surgery is to "teach, train and inspire excellence in students, residents, health care providers, and patients, with care and respect; to promote innovative, high-quality patient care; engage in cutting-edge research that enhances patient outcomes; and to contribute to the economic health of the University, the Medical Center, city and region."[37] As one of the founding departments of the Tulane University School of Medicine, the Department of Surgery has a long and illustrious history. The department is one of the oldest academic surgical departments in the United States. Since its earliest years, graduates of the Department of Surgery have become leaders in many surgical fields, and the number of "firsts" from Tulane faculty and residents is evidence of this.

Dr. Thomas Hunt, Dr. John H. Harrison, and Dr. Warren Stone founded the Medical College of Louisiana in 1834, and it later became Tulane University School of Medicine.

On September 29 of that year, the announcement of the opening of the college, as well as *The First Circular or Prospectus*

---

37 Tulane University, "Vision and Mission Statements," http://tulane.edu/som/departments/surgery/medical-education/general-surgery/vision-mission.cfm (accessed July 1, 2010).

of the Medical College of Louisiana, was published on the front page of *L'Abeille* (the *Bee*), New Orleans's most widely circulated newspaper of the time, which was printed in both French and English. Drs. Hunt, Harrison, and Stone drafted the prospectus six days earlier, and it outlined the considerations behind the decision to found a medical school in New Orleans:

1. Because it is the largest and most populous town in the South West, and the most accessible to students.

2. Because its Hospitals which will be open to the undersigned for the purpose of instruction are the largest in the Southern and Western States: so that practical Medicine and Surgery can be taught at the bedside of the patient—the only proper place for their study.

3. Because the study of Anatomy can be prosecuted with more advantage, and at a cheaper rate here than in any other city in the United States.

4. Because N.O. is so healthy during eight months in the year that students can remain in it, and study the different types of disease at different seasons.

5. Because it is a commercial town, and more surgical accidents occur to seamen than to any other class of individuals, and it is consequently the best field for the study of Surgery in the South West.

6. Because in consequence of its great population its hospitals are always filled with patients.

7. Because, as the undersigned pledge themselves, students can get board at $25 a month.[38]

The seven individuals who would comprise the faculty of the new institution signed the prospectus: Thomas Hunt, professor of anatomy and physiology; John H. Harrison, adjunct; Charles. A. Luzenberg, professor of principles and practice of surgery; J. Munro Mackie, professor of theory and practice of medicine; Thomas. R. Ingalls, professor of chemistry; Edwin Balhurst Smith, professor of materia medica; and Augustus H. Cenas, professor of obstetrics and diseases of women and children.

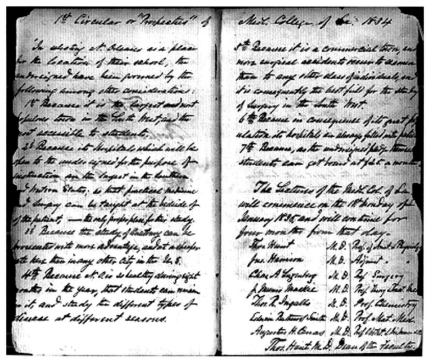

The prospectus as it appeared in *L'Abeille* in 1834.

38 Tulane University, "The Prospectus: Images of the Original Document and Verbatim Typescript," http://www.tulane.edu/~matas/historical/SpecColl/prospectus/prospectus_typed.htm (accessed July 29, 2010).

The standards for instruction at the school were typical of other medical institutions of the day, although graduation did not necessarily require a thorough knowledge of medicine. Initially, requirements for graduation included attendance of two full courses of lectures and one year of experience in a doctor's office. Four years of apprenticeship with a doctor was accepted in lieu of one course of lectures. The school year itself was only four months long, from December to March.[39]

The announcement of the new school created a storm of controversy among the *Bee*'s readership and in the medical community in New Orleans. The city's Creole physicians, many of whom had been educated in university settings in France, voiced concern about a medical school unattached to a university and the youthfulness of the new institution's founders (the oldest of whom was only twenty-six). Furthermore, the Creoles were concerned that the new English physicians would try to run them out of town and practice substandard medicine. They especially disapproved of the English physicians' liberal use of bloodletting.[40] Nevertheless, the school opened in January 1835, and Dr. Hunt delivered the first lecture in the Strangers Unitarian Church at St. Charles Avenue and Gravier Street. Initially, professors taught classes in a variety of locations, including Charity Hospital, which had been founded in 1736.

---

39 John Duffy, *The Tulane University Medical Center: One Hundred and Fifty Years of Medical Education* (Baton Rouge: Louisiana State University Press, 1984).
40 Ibid.

Charles Aloysius Luzenberg, 1835–1837

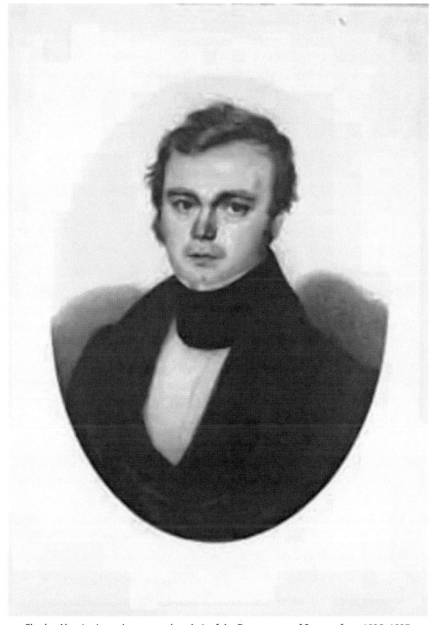

Charles Aloysius Luzenberg served as chair of the Department of Surgery from 1835–1837.

As one of the seven signers of the prospectus for the Medical College of Louisiana, Dr. Charles A. Luzenberg was the first professor of principles and practice of surgery at the school. Following the initial course of lectures in the spring of 1835 and the application for a charter, Dr. Luzenberg, along with professor of materia medica Dr. Edward H. Barton, drew up the school's constitution and bylaws. The constitution established seven chairs within the medical school, and the bylaws established procedures for faculty appointments and dismissals, the schedule of lectures, and course fees.

The medical community throughout the region recognized Luzenberg's surgical accomplishments. In 1830, Luzenberg was the second Louisiana physician to perform a cesarean section. That summer, a slave owner called in Luzenberg to perform the surgery after the in utero baby of one of his slaves had already been dead for several days. Luzenberg performed the procedure, but unfortunately the patient did not survive, having been severely ill before the procedure.[41] A New Orleans newspaper carried a report of an operation conducted by Dr. Luzenberg during the mid-1830s that involved "tying the carotid artery, and extirpating a sacromatous parotid gland, involving the ear and a large portion of the integuments of the cheek and neck." This surgery made him a local star and was a factor in Luzenberg's election to the Academy of Medicine of Paris. In 1834, Luzenberg performed the first successful ligation of the common iliac artery for aneurysm performed at Charity Hospital, where he served on the board of administrators for many years.[42]

Luzenberg founded the Franklin Infirmary in 1834, which was recognized as one of the best private hospitals in the area. Despite initial criticism by the local press, the hospital opened during the summer of 1835. Located in the Franklin district, from which the hospital derived its name, it accommodated

---

41 John Duffy (ed.), *The Rudolph Matas History of Medicine in Louisiana*, vol. 2 (Baton Rouge: Louisiana State University Press, 1962).
42 Ibid.

one hundred patients on three floors. The first floor was "for the better order of patients" and cost three dollars per day, the second floor cost one dollar per day, and the third floor was for the care of slaves. The hospital also provided medical students "an excellent opportunity of becoming practically conversant with their profession by placing themselves under the tuition of Dr. Luzenberg and attendings at his hospital."[43] This was an interesting contrast from Charity Hospital at that time. Of the 2,480 patients admitted to Charity in 1832, one-quarter died. Critics said that it was in part due to the poor nutrition that they received. At the time, one-fifth of the budget went to alcohol for the patients. In 1832, Charity used 749 gallons of Teneriffe wine, 12 hogsheads of claret, 1,306 gallons of whiskey, 102 gallons of rum, 6 gallons of gin, 3 gallons of brandy, and 48 containers of port wine.[44]

Following the resignation of Dr. Thomas Hunt as dean of the medical college in May 1835, Dr. Luzenberg was elected to replace him. Dr. Luzenberg's colleagues recognized his professional accomplishments. However, his brief tenure as a faculty member and as dean of the school was marked by a series of clashes with his fellow professors and the New Orleans medical community. In his history of the Tulane University Medical Center, John Duffy described Luzenberg as "a man of undoubted talents, but…also a prima donna of the first order."[45] Others described Luzenberg as "abrupt in speech, uncouth in manners, irritable and petulant in temper, and arrogant and overbearing in demeanor."[46]

One quarrel involving Dr. Luzenberg occurred when the faculty decided to change his course, Principles and Practice of Surgery, into Anatomy and Operative Surgery during a May 1836 meeting. Luzenberg refused to instruct the revised

---

43 Ibid.
44 John Salvaggio, *New Orleans' Charity Hospital: A Story of Physicians, Politics, and Poverty* (Baton Rouge: Louisiana State University Press, 1992).
45 Duffy, *The Tulane University Medical Center*, p. 12.
46 Ibid.

course, and two months later at a July 30 meeting the original course was reinstated. However, at the same meeting, the department replaced Luzenberg as dean with Dr. Barton. Following his replacement, Luzenberg refused to provide Barton items belonging to the office of the dean, including the college seal and the diploma plate. The department appointed a committee to resolve the matter, and it presumably was.[47]

Animosity between Luzenberg and Dr. Warren Stone, one of the founders of the medical college, was likely the cause behind Luzenberg's resignation from the school on January 28, 1837, and the appointment of Stone as the surgical chair. Prior to Luzenberg's resignation, students of the college had written a letter praising Dr. Stone. The letter, which also urged his appointment as professor of anatomy and operative surgery, was a response to a rumor that students were dissatisfied with Stone's teaching.

It is not documented whether Luzenberg was behind the rumor, but acrimony between the two men was known.

The memoirs of Dr. F.J.B. Romer, who was a resident and later assistant surgeon at Charity Hospital, illustrated one cause of Luzenberg's feelings toward Stone. Upon examining a man admitted to one of the wards at Charity, Luzenberg diagnosed him as having a malignant tumor, "probably a fungus hoematodes"—likely known today as retinoblastoma. Luzenberg returned later that evening with medical colleagues to discuss the case, only to find that Stone, unaware of Luzenberg's previous diagnosis, had examined the patient, found him to be suffering from an abscess, and opened it.[48]

Luzenberg's disagreements with others in the medical community continued after his resignation from the Medical College of Louisiana. The following year, he was involved in a scandal that received press throughout the United States. An April 1838 article entitled "Sight Given to the Born Blind" in the *True*

---

47 Ibid.
48 Ibid, p. 14.

American detailed an operation performed by Dr. Luzenberg on the eyes of a female Seminole patient. The reporter and author of the article, Charles J. B. Fisher, apparently embellished his story. A committee appointed by the Physico-Medical Society, the premier medical society in New Orleans at the time, to examine the case found that the woman was not blind, but only suffering from cataracts. The committee's finding that the operation resulted in the woman having greater impairment in one eye and losing the other eye completely was further damaging to Dr. Luzenberg. The committee also charged Luzenberg with knowingly permitting the embellished account to be published. The society expelled Luzenberg and resolved to notify the national medical community of its findings.[49]

Luzenberg vociferously denied the charges and even challenged the society's members to a series of duels, which he published in local newspapers. No duels actually occurred, but a fellow doctor returned Luzenberg's challenges with an advertisement that read in part "If that contemptible puppy, Charles A. Luzenberg...as at all anxious to enjoy the privilege of a shot he can obtain one by applying to:–J.S. McFarlane, Corner Poydras and Circus Sts. No substitutes admitted."[50] In addition to the physical threats, Luzenberg also accused a former colleague at the medical college of financial defrauding him.

His continued public pronouncements against other doctors in the area led the Physico-Medical Society to publish a pamphlet, which was circulated nationally, on the event and every other scandal associated with Luzenberg. The pamphlet also contained a statement by Dr. John J. Ker that stated that Luzenberg's preparations for duels included the suspension of "bodies of person who had died under his care whilst House

---

49 Duffy, *The Rudolph Matas History of Medicine in Louisiana.*
50 Ibid, p. 15.

Surgeon of the Charity Hospital" for target practice. Luzenberg never officially denied this accusation.[51]

Surprisingly, or not, these were not the only duel-inducing controversies at that time. Dr. Hunt, founder of the medical school, publicly criticized the political ideals of the *Crescent* newspaper editor, J. W. Frost. Frost subsequently challenged Hunt to a duel, and the two men met on the south side of the city and fired shotguns at each other on July 9, 1851. Hunt's second round wounded Frost in the chest, and he died the next day. Hunt left town for a few days but later surrendered himself to authorities and was released on ten-thousand-dollars bail. All the judges in the city refused to sit for the trial, and the district attorney dismissed the case since there was no one to try it.[52]

In 1856, two Charity surgeons, Dr. Samuel Choppin and Dr. John Foster, came to duels in the Charity courtyard. Their quarrel surrounded the right of who should care for a medical student named Mr. Weems. Mr. Weems had been shot by a law student at a Mardi Gras ball. Choppin and Foster began arguing at a dying Weems's bedside and had a "severe first encounter" that spilled into the Charity courtyard—luckily, both physicians missed. Three years later Choppin and Foster once again quarreled over the rights to treat a man with a carotid aneurysm. Their exchange is as follows:

> "Are you looking at me, sir?" asked Choppin, and Foster replied, "Yes, sir, I am looking at you." "And what do you think of me?" continued Choppin. Foster responded, "I think you are a God-damned scoundrel." At that instant, both physicians drew their pistols.

---

51 The pamphlet was entitled *Proceedings of the Physico-Medical Society of New Orleans, in Relation to the Trial and Expulsion of Charles A. Luzenberg, (With Comments by the Same)* (New Orleans, LA: Published by Order of the Society, 1838).

52 Duffy, *The Rudolph Matas History of Medicine in Louisiana.*

Foster shot Choppin through the neck with his self-cocking five-barrel revolver, shearing his jugular vein, and in the hip before Choppin could even cock his single barrel derringer. Choppin responded by charging Foster with a Bowie knife, at which point medical students stormed both men and broke up the fight. Choppin miraculously survived, and did not press charges against his old rival.[53]

Even with the aforementioned controversies, Luzenberg still maintained his supporters and was seemingly well regarded by patients. Thus, he remained in New Orleans until just before his death in 1848. This combination of medical acumen and a strong personality would actually become a hallmark of chairs of the surgery department at Tulane.

53 Salvaggio, *New Orleans' Charity Hospital.*

Warren Stone, 1837–1872

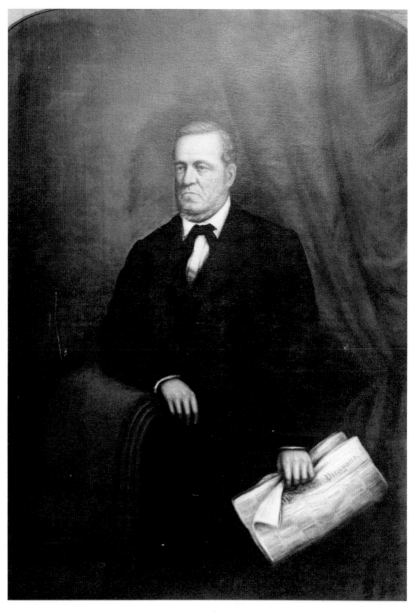

Warren Stone served as chair of the Department of Surgery from 1837–1872.

As mentioned previously, the resignation of Luzenberg as professor of surgery resulted in the election of Warren Stone to that position on January 28, 1837. While Stone assisted in the foundation of the medical college, he was not one of the original faculty during the first session. Rather, he served as the demonstrator of anatomy, then adjunct to the chair of anatomy and physiology. In addition to serving as chair of surgery from 1837 to 1872, Stone also served as chair of anatomy from 1837 to 1839. His reputation as a surgeon was known in New Orleans and throughout the nation.

Raised on a poor family farm in Vermont, Warren Stone attended the Medical School of Pittsfield, Massachusetts, before beginning his career in Troy, New York, in 1831. Two years later, Stone decided that New Orleans offered opportunities to advance his career. En route, the ship he was traveling on was beached and quarantined due to a cholera outbreak onboard. Stone assisted in the treatment of the victims, and while there met Dr. Thomas Hunt, and a strong friendship was quickly formed. This was a crucial relationship, paramount to the founding of the Medical College of Louisiana.[54]

Upon arriving in New Orleans in December 1833, Stone, almost penniless, secured a position at Charity Hospital from Hunt, eventually becoming assistant house surgeon. Working together, the two eventually met John Harrison and began to form the medical school. Hunt was known as the strong moving force, Stone was known as the "doer" of the operation, and Harrison was the more scholarly of the three.[55]

Stone's aforementioned experience treating cholera and yellow fever served him well in the Crescent City, where just two years earlier, both diseases had been widespread. Dr. Stone was likely the first physician to use quinine in the treatment of yellow fever, preferring it over the use of calomel. In Rudolph Matas's history of medicine in Louisiana, he reports that Stone

---

54 Ibid.
55 Duffy, *The Tulane University Medical Center.*

may have also been the first to use an intravenous saline mixture infusion in treating dehydration from Asiatic cholera while in New York in 1832. Stone did discover the benefit of cold water, used internally and externally, for cholera patients while treating patients at Charity Hospital in 1833.[56]

According to historian John Duffy, Dr. Stone "epitomized the nineteenth-century surgeon."[57] A large man, both physically and intellectually, he exhibited a ruggedness that sometimes dispensed with niceties. Given the nature of nineteenth-century surgery, this is not surprising. The grandmother of one young man contemplating instruction from Dr. Stone was informed "if...your grandson is timid, I doubt if he would profit much by Doctor Stone's tuition."[58] *Harper's Weekly* did a piece on Stone describing an amputation: "with cuffs thrown back, eye all ablaze, and lips firmly clinched, he prepares to make the adroit thrust...the sudden flash of polished steel; the dull, muffled sound of the yielding flesh, the spirt of blood... the sharp cry of the patient...these are the outlines of a picture that thrills and terrifies the uninitiated beholder."

Nonetheless, Dr. Stone's skills as a surgeon were well regarded to the point that Dr. Rudolph Matas considered him "probably Louisiana's greatest ante bellum surgeon."[59]

Dr. Stone performed the first successful amputation of the thigh under Letheon, or sulphuric ether, in Louisiana in February 1847. Alexander J. Wedderburn, professor of anatomy and clinical surgery at the Medical College of Louisiana and visiting surgeon of Charity Hospital, performed the second two months later.

Dr. Stone's work in the area of arterial surgery is most noteworthy. In 1859, he was the first to apply a silver ligature to an artery. Contrary to the common practice of the day, Stone also insisted the ligature not be drawn too tightly so as not to

---

56 Duffy, *The Rudolph Matas History of Medicine in Louisiana*, p. 20–21.
57 Duffy, *The Tulane University Medical Center*, p. 35.
58 Ibid, p. 35.
59 Duffy, *The Rudolph Matas History of Medicine in Louisiana*, p. 11.

injure the artery. Although the patient died within the month due to dysentery, the operation was of importance according to Dr. Matas because it marked "an original effort to advance the progress of arterial surgery."[60] Stone's efforts in the treatment of wounds and aneurysms of the gluteal artery were also credited to his skill as a surgeon.

In 1842, the faculty of the medical college petitioned the Louisiana legislature to make available land for the establishment of a medical school building. In March of the next year, a law was passed leasing to the school a lot at the corner of Philippa and Common Streets for ten years. In return, the faculty would care for the Charity patients free of charge. This began the first official relationship between the medical school and Charity Hospital. In fact, the faculty of the medical school provided care to the Charity patients free of charge until the 1960s. A three-story building that contained a lecture room large enough for two hundred students, a chemical laboratory, two smaller rooms intended to serve as a library and reading room, and a dissecting room was the first permanent home for the school, occupied in 1844. The cost of the building at that time was fifteen thousand dollars.[61]

Dr. Stone oversaw the transition of the Medical College of Louisiana into the Medical Department of the University of Louisiana in 1847, established because of the land grant by the Louisiana legislature. By the end of 1847, the medical department relocated to a building on Common Street between Baronne and Philippa, which was described as one of the largest medical school buildings in the country. [62]

60 Ibid, p. 51.
61 Salvaggio. *New Orleans' Charity Hospital.*
62 Duffy, *The Tulane University Medical Center.*

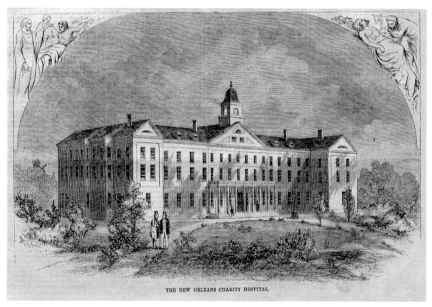

Charity Hospital as it appeared circa 1833.

Many of the clinical experiences for students took place at Charity Hospital. In 1859, Charity was the largest hospital in the world, admitting 12,775 patients, and had the fourth-largest medical school in the country. However, like much of New Orleans, the medical school was greatly affected by the Civil War, closing on November 2, 1863, and remaining shuttered until November 1865. Charity remained open but operated under a severe shortage of physicians and personnel after federal troops occupied the city and took control of the hospital.[63] The years following the war were difficult for the institution as it sought to rebuild after neglect and the dispersal of its faculty and students. Dr. Stone took the first step in returning medical education to New Orleans when he announced on January 13, 1865, that he would present lectures on practical surgery twice a week at the university. The school would not open until the

---

63 Salvaggio, *New Orleans' Charity Hospital*.

following November, and there is no evidence as to whether the lectures took place. However, Stone was one of the faculty attending an October 1865 meeting to discuss reopening the school.[64]

Stone continued to serve as chair of surgery until April 30, 1872, when he submitted his resignation. He passed away later that year.

Tobias Gibson Richardson, 1872–1889

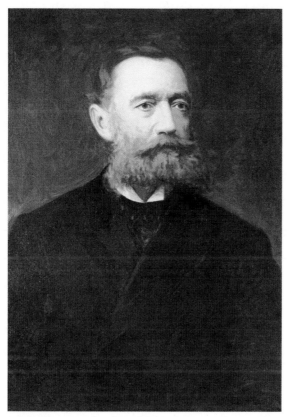

Tobias Gibson Richardson served as chair of the Department of Surgery from 1872–1889.

---

64 Duffy, *The Tulane University Medical Center.*

Dr. Tobias G. Richardson succeeded Dr. Stone as chair of surgery in the medical school. Dr. Richardson received his medical training in Louisville, Kentucky, and later served on the faculty of the University of Louisville and the Jefferson Medical College in Philadelphia before journeying to New Orleans. He would be the first chair of the department with formal surgery training. His *Elements of Human Anatomy* was published in 1854 and remained a standard textbook in Southern medical schools for many years. Dr. Richardson joined the faculty at the University of Louisiana as professor of anatomy in 1858. He was the first to perform an amputation of both legs at the hip in which the patient made a complete recovery. He served as chief surgeon to the Confederate Army of Tennessee during the Civil War, and when the school reopened in 1865, Richardson was elected as dean of the school, a position he held until 1885. He also was the first doctor from Louisiana to serve as president of the American Medical Association, a position he held from 1877–1878. There have been a total of three doctors from Louisiana to serve as president of the AMA, one in each century. Donald J. Palmisano, MD, JD, FACS, a graduate of Tulane School of Medicine and a Tulane surgery residency graduate, is the most recent (2003–2004).

Dr. Richardson oversaw the school during very difficult years following the war. In 1872, Samuel Logan replaced Richardson as the chair of anatomy, and Richardson became the chair of surgery. However, ten years later, Richardson asked to be relieved of his professorship of surgery due to the lack of surgical cases at Charity Hospital. In his complaint, Dr. Richardson stated that his wards had not "an amputation, dislocation, or other complicated case, and [he] had seen only three patients with fractures."[65]

The issue of the distribution of surgical and medical cases had been an ongoing issue among professors of the medical school. In this instance, Richardson sent a letter to the medi-

---

65 Ibid., p. 59.

cal school faculty and to Charity Hospital stating that Samuel Logan, as professor of anatomy and clinical surgery, received better cases, to which Dr. Logan replied that if such was the case, it was due to the superior ability of his resident students. Ultimately, a compromise was reached that allowed the professors of clinical surgery and surgery to use cases at Charity under the care of any faculty member to illustrate lectures.

During Dean Richardson's tenure, the medical school transitioned from the University of Louisiana to Tulane University following a large donation by philanthropist Paul Tulane in 1882. The University of Louisiana then became Tulane University of Louisiana. Paul Tulane's $1.25 million donation transitioned the school from a largely state-supported to a now private entity.

Throughout the years, as medical training itself developed, surgical training at the medical school expanded. By 1880, the school year had expanded by six weeks. The first three weeks of the term were devoted exclusively to clinical medicine and surgery. In 1886, Tulane established its first premedical course. The professor of general and clinical surgery and the professor of anatomy and clinical surgery regularly held lectures at Charity Hospital. Finally, in 1907, in an attempt to increase the quality of medical education and physicians across the country, medical schools nationwide required a high school diploma for admission.[66]

The schedule of weekly didactic lectures for each department as listed in the medical school catalogue for 1884/1885 provides a glimpse of the topics addressed. Topics for the surgical lectures were held in this order: causes and treatment of acute inflammation; chronic inflammation; tumors benign and malignant; injuries—constitutional and local effects, contusions, and wounds; hemorrhage; injuries of arteries, veins, and nerves; injuries of bones—contusions and fractures; injuries of joints—contusions, wounds, dislocations; diseases of

66 Ibid.

bones and joints; and erysipelas, burns, and tetanus. These were followed by lectures on regional surgery in the following areas: head; face and throat; cervical region; thorax and abdomen; and pelvis.

After serving thirty-two years on the faculty of the medical school, Dr. Richardson resigned in May 1889 due to poor health. His wife, Ida, later provided the donations that aided the construction of the Richardson Building on Canal Street, which housed the medical school, and other buildings on Tulane's campus.[67] In 1893, the School of Medicine moved to the Richardson Building on Canal Street for their training. It would be later named the Hutchinson Building, and a new building on Tulane's uptown campus would be named the Richardson Building to keep the memory of the generous donations from the Richardsons alive.

As stated in Dr. Richardson's aforementioned letter, an emphasis on clinical training at Charity Hospital and other institutions was an integral part of instruction at the school. Although the hospital had been utilized as a location for classes since the very first term of the Medical College of Louisiana, the act that established the University of Louisiana in 1847 gave the faculty of the medical department use of Charity for practical instruction. Echoing the initial prospectus for the school, a later prospectus specifically cited Charity's role in surgical education in New Orleans:

> In the Surgical Department, the advantages of this College rank those of all others in the Union. The number of wounds, fractures, dislocations, and other injuries, and disease requiring the frequent exercise of Operative Surgery, admitted into the Wards of the New Orleans Hospital, will

---

67 Ibid.

be found on examination to exceed that of any other in America.[68]

As early as the 1870s, the annual circular of the medical school also emphasized the importance of the hospital to medical training when it stated, "It is universally admitted that without abundant anatomical and clinical material, no medical school, however numerous or eloquent its professors, can possibly fit its pupils for practical professional life."[69] By 1884, fourteen of Charity's fifty-two wards were surgical wards. The professor of surgery visited the wards from nine to ten every morning and expected students to attend the wards at this time and "familiarize themselves at the bedside of the Patients, with the diagnosis and treatment of all forms of injury and disease."[70]

In 1893, the School of Medicine moved to the Richardson Building on Canal Street. The construction of the new Richardson Building on Canal Street in 1893 provided Tulane with one of the best-equipped medical buildings in the nation. In addition to larger classrooms, laboratories for chemistry, pharmacy, practical anatomy, microscopical anatomy, pathology, and bacteriology were available. The school added an operative surgery course, which was taught in the Laboratory of Practical Anatomy. Taught by Dr. Warren S. Bickham, demonstrator of operative surgery, the course was obligatory for graduation, and students could obtain certificates of attendance for one dollar. The 1893/1894 catalogue described the course thus:

> The entire field of General Surgery will be gone over, the steps of each operation being first admirably

68 Douglas R. Lincoln, "The History of Tulane University School of Medicine's Involvement with Charity Hospital," http://www.tulane.edu/~matas/historical/charity/charity3.htm (accessed July 15, 2010).

69 *Annual Circular of the Medical Department of the University of Louisiana for the Session 1879–'80 and Catalogue of the Graduating Class of Session 1878–'79*, p. 3

70 *Announcement of the University of Louisiana, 1884–85. Catalogue of the Academical Department, Sixth Session, 1883–1884* (New Orleans, G. T. Lathrop, Printer, 1884), p. 2.

illustrated by means of an Electric Optical Projector, and fully explained by the Demonstrator, after which the students, in sections, will perform the operations in the presence of the Demonstrator and the class.[71]

Another bequest, in 1902, from Alexander Charles Hutchinson allowed for the renovation and renaming of the Richardson Building. The department organized and equipped a Laboratory of Minor Surgery, which aimed to prepare students for later work in the surgical clinics at Charity Hospital. It included a systematic course of demonstrations and individual exercises in minor surgical procedures, including first aid to the injured and in emergencies. The course consisted of three demonstrations per week for first-year students and one weekly demonstration in more advanced studies and procedures for second-year students.

This major renovation also resulted in the addition of the Hutchinson Clinics, and the building was renamed the Josephine Hutchinson Memorial Building. One of the additional buildings constructed on Tulane's uptown campus and financed by the Hutchinson gift was named the Richardson Memorial Building in order to continue the tribute to former Dean Richardson at Tulane.[72]

The Hutchinson donation occurred just prior to the expansion of the medical school curriculum to a four-year program, which required additional space for the medical school. Thus, from 1907 until 1963, first- and second-year students were taught in the Richardson Memorial Building uptown before continuing their studies downtown.

Tulane medical students would also play an important part in the city in 1914. Doctors diagnosed two immigrants with bubonic plague, and panic soon ensued throughout the city. People at that time knew that rats spread the disease, and not

71 Tulane University of Louisiana, *Catalogue 1893–94* (New Orleans: Tulane University of Louisiana, 1894), p. 135.
72 Duffy, *The Tulane University Medical Center.*

surprisingly, New Orleans had a very healthy rat population. The city organized rat patrols, consisting of Tulane medical students, to collect rats and dissect them looking for signs of the plague. The Tulane rat-collection program was so robust that it was thought that the medical students killed nearly one-third of New Orleans's rat population. They also injected horses with the plague found in the rats to create "anti-serum" and saved several of the infected patients.[73]

Although the medical department had allowed its graduates to attend clinical courses for a number of years, in 1906 the Tulane School of Medicine took steps to add graduate education to its curriculum by integrating the New Orleans Polyclinic and making it the postgraduate medical department. Founded in 1888, the Polyclinic was the third-oldest postgraduate school of medicine in the United States. From its early years, the two medical institutions maintained a cooperative relationship, with only minor issues arising from time to time.[74]

At the time of the integration, the Polyclinic faculty consisted of twenty-one professors and twenty-six lecturers and assistants, and a number of its staff also held appointments at the medical school. Initially, courses included general surgery, operative and clinical surgery, and clinical and minor surgery. However, when the medical department was reorganized as the College of Medicine in 1913, graduate training expanded. By the 1930s, added courses covered abdominal surgery, industrial surgery, urology, and orthopedics and surgical diseases of children. The Polyclinic was eventually renamed the Graduate School of Medicine and continued to operate as a separate unit within the college until it was fully absorbed and renamed the Division of Graduate Medicine. Following the integration of Graduate School of Medicine into the School of Medicine in 1937, postgraduate offerings within the Department of Surgery expanded to include courses in general surgery, plastic surgery,

73 Duffy, *The Rudolph Matas History of Medicine in Louisiana.*
74 Duffy, *The Tulane University Medical Center.*

and neurosurgery that included three years' residence, as well as fellowships and long courses that required one years' residence. These courses would evolve into the surgery residency program.[75]

Samuel Logan, 1889–1893

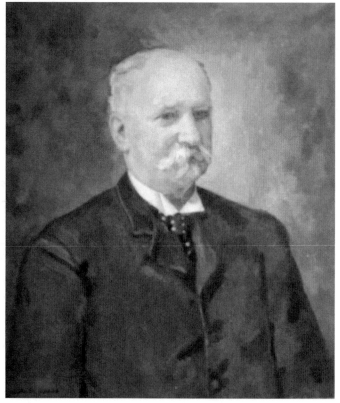

Samuel Logan served as chair of the Department of Surgery from 1889–1893.

Following the resignation of Dr. Richardson, two individuals during the next five years held the chair in surgery before Rudolph Matas assumed the position for more than thirty years.

75 Ibid.

Dr. Samuel Logan served as chair of surgery from 1889 to 1893. Formerly the dean of the short-lived New Orleans School of Medicine, Logan had joined the medical school faculty in the 1870s. His tumultuous relationship with Dr. Richardson was previously discussed; his time as chair was otherwise unremarkable. Following Dr. Logan's death in January 1893, Dr. Albert B. Miles succeeded him as chair of surgery for a year prior to his death from hemorrhagic typhoid fever in 1894.

Albert Baldwin Miles, 1893–1894

Born in Prattville, Alabama, in 1852, Dr. Miles studied medicine at Tulane before being elected house surgeon at Charity Hospital in 1882. During his association with Charity, Miles designed the buildings for two clinics connected with the hospital, which opened in April 1892, and supported the establishment of the Charity Hospital Training School for nurses. While at Tulane and Charity, Dr. Miles was a vocal advocate for the erection of a new surgical amphitheater at the hospital that would largely be used by Tulane students and faculty. Supported largely by Charity with contributions by Tulane faculty and (reluctantly) the university board of administrators, the A. B. Miles Surgical Amphitheatre was completed in 1895 and was furnished with "modern surgical and electrical appliances," according to the opening announcement. Following his death, Miles's will left ten thousand dollars to the medical department, which assisted the medical school library and helped establish a Miles Studentship that awarded the recipient free tuition and the ability to live in the hospital.[76]

---

76 Ibid.

Rudolph Matas, 1895–1927

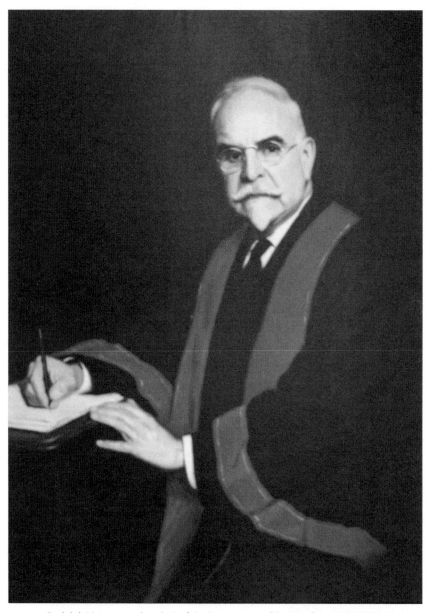

Rudolph Matas served as chair of the Department of Surgery from 1895–1927.

The death of Dr. Miles and the election of Rudolph Matas as the head of surgery in 1895 reflect the transformation in medicine and medical training from the nineteenth century into the twentieth century, not only within the surgical arena but also within the medical school as a whole. In his history of the Tulane Medical Center, John Duffy states that until the 1900s, the history of the medical school was "largely the history of the occupants of the seven professorial chairs."[77] In 1910, due to the merger of the New Orleans Polyclinic (which had become the postgraduate medical department at Tulane in 1906) with the medical department and the addition of dental and tropical medicine departments, the medical school was reorganized into eight major teaching divisions, of which surgery was one. Three years later, the nomenclature of the school was changed to the College of Medicine, which included the School of Medicine, the School of Pharmacy, the Graduate School of Medicine, and the School of Dentistry.[78]

Overseeing these changes and their effects on surgical training at Tulane, Dr. Rudolph Matas chaired the Department of Surgery for thirty-two years from 1895 to 1927. Considered by many to be Tulane's most distinguished medical alumnus, the medical community recognized Dr. Matas as the "Father of Vascular Surgery," and Sir William Osler hailed him as "that modern Antyllus" in 1915. When Matas started around 1881, doctors treated 96 percent of all hospital cases at Charity medically. That year, the 172 total surgical procedures included 72 amputations, 32 drained abscesses, 3 ligated arteries, 18 projectile extractions, and only one single laparotomy. Forty years later, at the end of Matas's time, nearly 80 percent of patients entering Charity would undergo a surgical intervention.[79]

A native of Louisiana, Matas was born in Bonnett Carre, Louisiana, in 1860 during the Civil War. He was born on a plantation where his father, a native from Spain, had been

77 Ibid., p. 107.
78 In 1932, the College of Medicine was renamed the School of Medicine.
79 Salvaggio, *New Orleans' Charity Hospital.*

hired to be the physician for the slaves. He entered the University of Louisiana medical school at the age of seventeen and graduated at the age of nineteen, after spending much of his youth in Barcelona, Paris, and Matamoras, Mexico. In fact, officials at first denied his admission because they did not believe he was native to Louisiana, being fluent in multiple languages at such a young age.[80] Much later in his career, he was noted for giving a welcome address in English, Spanish, French, and then Italian—all with no notes. As a student at Tulane, Dean Stanford E. Chaillé asked Matas to accompany a Yellow Fever Commission to Cuba. While there, he met Cuban physician Carlos Finlay, who first suggested the *Culex* mosquito as the transmitter of yellow fever. Matas translated Finlay's controversial paper on the subject in the *New Orleans Medical and Surgical Journal* in February 1882, which later won him an award from the Cuban government.[81] At 21, Dr Matas became editor of the *New Orleans Medical and Surgical Journal*, which was the oldest Southern medical periodical. Despite his young age, few questioned the wisdom of this decision.[82]

---

80 Roger Gregory, "Rudolph Matas—How I Remember Him: An Interview with Dr. Michael E. DeBakey," *J Vasc Surg* 34 (2001):384–86.
81 Salvaggio, *New Orleans' Charity Hospital.*
82 John Ochsner, "The Complex Life of Rudolph Matas," *J Vasc Surg* 34 (2001):387–92.

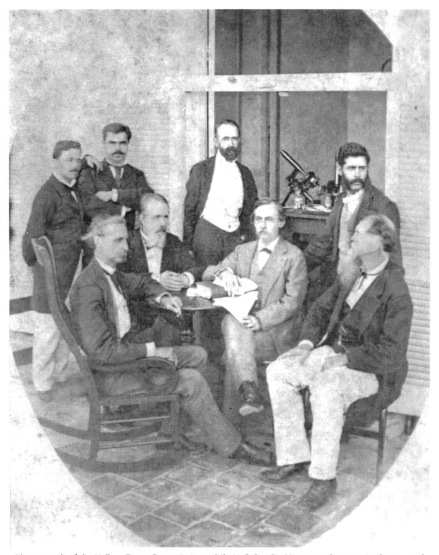

Photograph of the Yellow Fever Commission while in Cuba. Dr. Matas can be seen in the second row, second from the left.

Prior to Matas joining the faculty of his alma mater, he served as demonstrator of anatomy, as well as visiting surgeon and consulting surgeon of the eye, ear, nose, and throat at Charity Hospital, and was among the first to perform a thyroidectomy.[83] Matas had made a name for himself at the age of 28 in 1888 when he performed the first operation of endoaneurysmorrhaphy on a patient with a traumatic aneurysm of the brachial artery after being hit by a machete in the sugarcane fields of Louisiana. Matas first ligated the aneurysm proximally and distally, noting the next day that this still did not control the bleeding. He then decided to take the patient back to the operating room. He opened the aneurysm and noted collaterals in the wall of the sac that continued to leak into the lumen of the artery. After oversewing the walls, the bleeding and aneurysm were controlled.[84] According to Dr. Robert Hewitt, "[his] concept of obliteration or reconstruction from within the aneurysm was a monumental advance and is a principle that has endured and forms the basis of modern aneurysm repair."[85]

Matas also picked up Halstead's work with local anesthesia, being one of the first to perform upper and lower extremity amputations using a regional nerve block. Matas's accomplishments resulted in international awards and acclaim and included: surgery of the chest, abdomen, and blood vessels; his development of the intravenous drip technique; pulmonary insuflation; suction drainage in abdominal operations; operating under spinal anesthesia; surgical correction of appendicitis; and many other accomplishments. Even more impressive is that fact that Matas was able to accomplish all this with only one eye. In his early days as a surgeon, he got contaminated pus in his eye while removing a tubal ovarian abscess and lost his right eye after contracting gonococcal conjunctivitis.[86]

---

83 Salvaggio, *New Orleans' Charity Hospital.*
84 Duffy, *The Tulane University Medical Center.*
85 Robert L. Hewitt, "An Austere Tradition: The Story of Medicine at Tulane," *Tulane Medicine* (Spring 1994), p. 13.
86 Ochsner, "The Complex Life of Rudolph Matas."

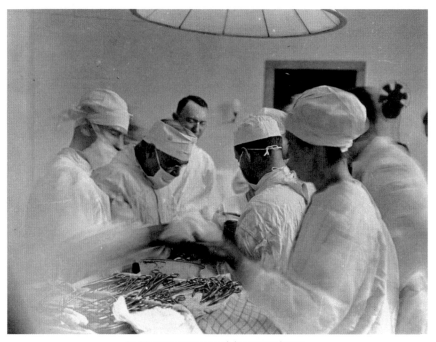

Dr. Matas operating with his surgical team.

Matas later went on to marry his longtime love, Adrienne Landry. She was the daughter of Captain Goslee of the Confederate Army, who was one of Dr. Matas's patients. When they first met in 1881, she was married to Arthur Landry, who later left her and their two children. Matas fell in love with her instantly while taking care of her father but waited patiently for nearly fifteen years.[87] Matas would make any excuse possible to see Adrienne and even hired her as a housekeeper. After Arthur and Adrienne's marriage was annulled by the Catholic Church, Matas married Adrienne in 1895 and adopted her two children. Sadly, Adrienne's only pregnancy with Matas ended in a stillbirth that was deeply devastating to Matas.[88]

87 Ibid.
88 Ibid.

Always known for his convivial nature and many friends, Matas also had two notable friendships throughout his professional career. They were Dr. William Mayo and Dr. William Halsted.[89] His close friendship with Halsted was fascinating, given Matas's outgoing nature and Halsted's famously withdrawn demeanor. Halsted and Matas frequently corresponded and visited each other's houses. On one such trip in 1903, Halsted secretly performed an orchiectomy on Matas for a right testicular seminoma, a secret that was not discovered until long after Matas's death in 1957. The orchiectomy was noted on his autopsy, but it was a mystery as to what had happened until correspondence between the two was found nearly half a century later in the 1990s.[90]

Like many of his predecessors, Dr. Matas's tenure was not without its controversy. In 1907, the Tulane board of administrators authorized an increase in four additional professorships in the medical school. They offered the chair in general and clinical surgery to Dr. F. W. Parham; however, Dr. Matas produced a resolution stating that additional chairs in clinical surgery should not affect his "official seniority…over the surgical laboratories and other intramural dependencies."[91] Although Matas withdrew his statement, Dr. Parham refused the offer from Tulane's medical school.

The following spring saw the acceptance of the physiology chair by Gustav Mann in March 1908, which would eventually provide additional issues for the Department of Surgery. Mann's 1915 Ivy Day speech was a culmination of his increasingly vocal dissatisfaction with the medical school and was seen as an attack on the school and on Dr. Matas and the Department of Surgery in particular. His comments focused on perceived inadequacies in the clinical aspect of surgery training

---

89 Roger Gregory, "Childhood Memories of Giants in Vascular Surgery: Matas, DeBakey, de Takats, and Ochsner. An Interview with Dr. John Ochsner," *Cardiovascular Surgery* 11 (2001):5, 407–11.
90 Daniel Nunn, "Dr. Halsted's Secret Operation on Dr. Matas." Presented at the 65th Annual Meeting of the Halsted Society, September 4, 1991.
91 Duffy, *The Tulane University Medical Center*, p. 104.

at Tulane and on the timeliness of Dr. Matas and others in the department.[92]

When Dr. Mann delivered his Ivy Day speech, his main point of contention was that third-year students could not understand what was occurring during surgery demonstrations as they lacked previous instruction in operative surgery. Beginning in 1907, the medical school catalogues provide the clearest views on the annual structure of surgical training at Tulane and show that Mann may not have been completely off in his comments.[93]

The first and second years of instruction included laboratories and courses in minor surgery. The first year included a minor surgery laboratory, while the second included two courses on surgery: a laboratory course in minor surgery on more advanced studies and a clinical course in the wards and in the out-clinics of the Charity Hospital. During the third year, a course in clinical surgery provided students training in recording cases, discussing surgical procedures, prognosis, diagnosis, and aftercare of surgical cases. Didactic lectures and demonstrations on surgical pathology and the principles of surgery were given at the Hutchinson Building. Dr. Matas gave clinical lectures in the hospital amphitheater on Mondays, Thursdays, and Saturdays, often where operations were performed before the class.[94]

During the students' final year, sections of the class received clinical instruction in the wards and at patient bedsides. Professors demonstrated the elements of asepsis and antisepsis, and the principles of surgical techniques and gave students the opportunity to assist in operations. In addition, Dr. Matas gave a weekly lecture on regional surgery, in addition to the course on operative surgery that has previously been discussed. Instruction included a course on genito-urinary and venereal diseases and assigned cases for students "for practice in the

92 Ibid.
93 Ibid.
94 Salvaggio, *New Orleans' Charity Hospital.*

examination of patients, passage of sounds, in irrigation methods, etc."[95]

During his Ivy Day speech, Dr. Mann also stated that many students graduated without having given anesthesia. This was not accurate because by 1909, Dr. Ansell M. Caine gave special instruction and demonstrations in the methods of general anesthesia at the surgical clinics and before class sections assigned to the surgery division. Dr. Caine was one of the founders of organized anesthesiology, and his instruction at Tulane continued through 1947.[96]

The following chart provides the distribution of instruction for students in the Department of Surgery for the 1912–1913 session, which provided a total of 814 hours of instruction.

	Laboratory	Lectures and recitations	Amphitheater	Clinics	Totals
Operative Surgery	90				90
Minor Surgery	45	15			60
General Surgery		90	165	104	359
Genito-Urinary Surgery		30		20	50
Orthopedics		30		20	50
Diseases of the Skin		55		30	85
Diseases of the Eye		35	15	20	70
Diseases of the Ear, Nose and Throat		30		20	50
				Grand Total	814

While there may have been a basis for Mann's comments in his 1915 Ivy Day speech, they nonetheless resulted in his dismissal.

95 *Bulletin of the Tulane University of Louisiana. Medical Department (Undergraduate), 1907–1908*, p. 38.

96 Salvaggio, *New Orleans' Charity Hospital*.

War again interrupted surgical training at Tulane—this time during World War I. At the same time, it provided the school and Dr. Matas with the ability to provide leadership in the area of medical preparedness. After the organization of a national committee on the topic, Dr. Matas served as the Louisiana representative. He also oversaw the formation of a base hospital equipped by the New Orleans chapter of the Red Cross and staffed by professors and students from Tulane. Established in 1916, the Tulane Unit, Base Hospital No. 24, eventually served with distinction in France. Considered essential to the school, Dr. Matas did not follow the hospital to Europe; he did, however, organize an "Officer's School for Instruction in War Fractures and Other Ward Wounds," which became one of four such schools for wartime trauma established by the US Surgeon General during the war.[97]

In this golden age of surgery, Dr. Matas mentored an array of young surgeons. One notable surgeon was Dr. Alberto Garcia. Dr. Garcia was born in Mexico in 1889 and later became a ward of Dr. John Harvey Kellogg (of Kellogg Corn Flakes fame) in Michigan at the age of ten. Garcia first received his medical degree from the American Medical Missionary College in 1910 but was admitted to Tulane School of Medicine in 1913 to earn his American medical degree. He then became the first Mexican to be trained in the United States in the modern medical era. At Tulane, he would go on to perform the first open heart surgery in Louisiana, operating on a young black man who was taken to Charity during Mardi Gras. His daughter, Dr. Maria Esperanza Garcia Roach, would later teach anesthesia at Charity Hospital beginning in 1940, working closely with Drs. DeBakey and Ochsner.

Dr. Matas reached Tulane's official retirement age in 1925. Over his lifetime, he amassed a large personal collection of books and was a devout student of history. He had acquired so many books in his 2255 St. Charles Ave. house that the foun-

---

97 Ochsner, "The Complex Life of Rudolph Matas."

dation had to be reinforced, and other physicians often sent students to fetch books from Matas's personal collection that the school library had not yet acquired. His St. Charles house became an institution for the surgical department throughout his tenure and even stayed open during his final years while he was hospitalized. His Mardi Gras parties were well attended, with the King of Mardi Gras always stopping the parade for a special toast to Matas.[98] Upon his death, he left his personal collection to Tulane—what has now become the Tulane Matas Library. By 1954, he was confined to a wheelchair and could no long see. The members of the local Nu Sigma Nu fraternity would take turns reading to him to help stem his insatiable thirst for knowledge—although it was well-known that he was quite a fan of the occasional trashy mystery novel. Matas spent the last three years of his life hospitalized, and the last eighteen months receiving nourishment through a feeding tube.[99] He died on September 23, 1958, at the age of 97.

---

98 Gregory, "Rudolph Matas—How I Remember Him."
99 Ochsner, "The Complex Life of Rudolph Matas."

Edward William Alton Ochsner, 1927–1956

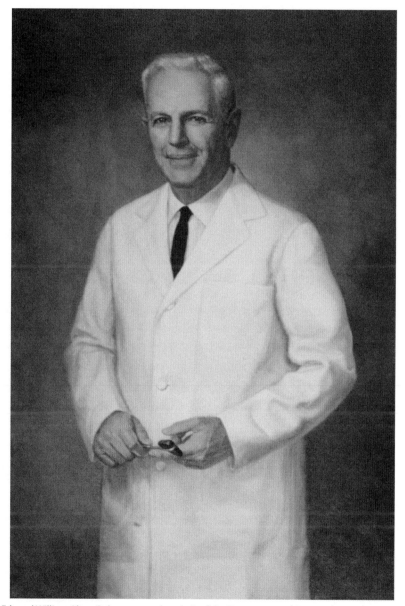

Edward William Alton Ochsner served as chair of the Department of Surgery from 1927–1956.

Following Dr. Matas's retirement, many believed Dr. Mims Gage, one of the surgery faculty, to be the most qualified internal candidate. Ultimately, those responsible for naming a new chair decided on an outside candidate. After a two-year search, they recruited thirty-one-year-old E. W. Alton Ochsner from the University of Wisconsin Medical School to head the Department of Surgery. Characteristic of New Orleans hospitality, Dr. Mims Gage developed a great friendship with Dr. Ochsner and even let him live at his home when he first arrived. Dr. Mims Gage's son is named John Ochsner Gage, MD, and one of Dr. Ochsner's sons, now deceased, was named Mims Gage Ochsner. Filling a position held by someone with the reputation of Dr. Matas would not be easy for anyone, and Ochsner was not only young, but also an outsider to the Tulane system. However, during his thirty-year tenure, Ochsner not only built a reputation as a determined teacher and leading surgeon, but would leave a legacy to New Orleans medicine with the establishment of the Ochsner Clinic.

Ochsner was born in Kimball, South Dakota, in 1896—the only son with five older sisters. Ochsner's uncle, A. J. Ochsner, was a famous surgeon at the University of Illinois at Chicago and best friends with William J. Mayo. He was a great help along Alton's career, including his admittance to Washington University Medical School in St. Louis. In 1922, Ochsner traveled to Europe for surgical training as many did at the time. He gained fame throughout Europe after orchestrating a series of successful blood transfusions in Switzerland. Blood transfusions had been done in Europe decades before but had not been successful due to many cross-reactions. Ochsner had learned how to type blood while working for his uncle the year after medical school in Chicago.[100] While in Switzerland, he was eager to prove that blood transfusions could be done successfully. He was first allowed to attempt transfusion on an inmate, which was successful. However, several days later, the president

---

100 Recording of Alton Ochsner distributed in 1999 by the Alton Ochsner Foundation.

of a large Swiss bank was admitted with severe blood loss from a bleeding ulcer. The Swiss doctors were unable to stabilize the patient and allowed Ochsner to perform a blood transfusion. Its success earned Ochsner instant respect throughout Europe.[101]

In 1923, while still in Switzerland, he married the daughter of a wealthy Chicago family. Upon his return to the United States, he quickly gained a position at the University of Wisconsin. In 1927, again thanks to the contacts of his uncle, he was offered the position of chair of the Tulane Department of Surgery.[102] He soon became famous in New Orleans for his quote, "early to bed, early to rise, work hard and publicize."

During his initial visit to the campus, Matas wanted to show off his surgical skills in a very spectacular manner. That day, Matas removed a 92-pound tumor from a 182-pound woman. It was so large, it had to be lifted out with a pulley system attached to the ceiling.[103] Ironically, the patient died the next day secondary to blood loss—as Tulane had not yet adopted the capability for blood transfusions.

Ochsner's interest and research in the area of lung cancer developed while a student at Washington University. Witnessing an autopsy of a patient who had died of carcinoma of the lung, Ochsner's professor told him that he may never see another such case. Ochsner recalled this when, years later while at Charity Hospital, he observed nine cases in a six-month period during 1936. His investigations and the determination that all the patients were heavy smokers led to Ochsner's early belief in the link between smoking and lung cancer.[104] Ochsner performed the first pneumonectomy in the Deep South on April 15, 1936, "as a means of dealing with a malignant bronchial lesion."[105]

101 Edward Haslam, *Dr. Mary's Monkey* (Walterville, OR: TrineDay, 2007).
102 Ibid.
103 Ibid.
104 Ochsner and colleague Michael DeBakey published a paper on the topic, "Primary Pulmonary Malignancy" in *Surgery, Gynecology and Obstetrics* 68 (1939): 433–51.
105 John Wilds and Ira Harkey, *Alton Ochsner: Surgeon of the South* (Baton Rouge: Louisiana State University, 1990), p. 181.

It is rumored that Ochsner even diagnosed King George VI's lung cancer after receiving his medical records from London.

Dr. Ochsner began Tulane's Interdepartmental Tumor Conference in 1940, and it eventually became the oldest multidisciplinary treatment planning tumor board in Louisiana. Designed as a consultative and educational conference for review of cancer cases at Tulane University Hospital and Tulane services at the Charity Hospitals in New Orleans, Independence, and Pineville, Louisiana, the conference convened weekly and was attended by faculty in the areas of diagnostic radiology, pathology, radiation oncology, surgical oncology, gynecologic oncology, and medical oncology, as well as students, interns, residents, allied health care providers, visiting cancer experts, and other interested professionals. During the conference sessions, medical practitioners presented patient cases for consultation and recommendations. Ochsner would go on to become the president of the American Cancer Society in 1949.

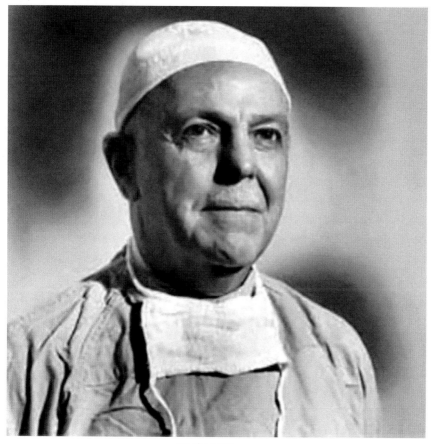

Dr. Alton Ochsner.

Not only was Ochsner a well-respected surgeon, but his influence on surgical training was an additional legacy. During his time at Tulane, Ochsner furthered Charity Hospital's role as a critical component in clinical surgical training. His use of the A. B. Miles Amphitheater as a "bullpen" where he grilled students and residents on their diagnoses was featured in a 1956 article in *Time.* They were so intense that one student even fainted when she was in the hot seat. Dr. Ochsner's efforts to teach students to work and think under pressure continued until the late 1970s. This training program continues to this day and is currently overseen by Dr. Bernard Jaffe.

In 1930, the School of Medicine moved from the old Hutchinson Building on Canal Street to a new Hutchinson Memorial Building on Tulane Avenue next to Charity Hospital—additional buildings were added in 1959 and 1963. To put things into perspective as to what running a surgical service at Charity was like, in 1935, the operating expenses for Charity were $1,358,054.12 for 67,952 inpatient visits and 473,986 outpatient visits. This broke down to $1.24 per inpatient day and $0.02 per outpatient visit. Further, the hospital's listed bed capacity was 1,814, but the actual census was usually around 2,781—with usually two and sometimes three patients to a bed. However, Ochsner's views of Charity and its usefulness to Tulane were not always favorable, and he seemingly had little patience for the role of politics at the hospital.[106]

In 1928, Huey P. Long, the "Kingfish," was elected governor of Louisiana. In his campaign he stated, "Huey P. Long…keenly appreciates the necessity of keeping the throttling hand of petty politics off the neck of this wonderful refuge of the sick…and he will not permit the efficient management of the hospital be subordinated to the ugly exigencies of partisan politics."[107] However, as one of his first acts as governor he removed as many board members as he could from Charity who did not support his campaign. He often politicized the Charity hospital system and was notorious for his nepotism to political supporters. In 1930, angry that Tulane did not have a say in choosing Charity residents and contemplating a move to head the surgery department at another school, Ochsner expressed his opinions regarding Charity in a letter to Allen Whipple, of Columbia Medical School. He stated, "the outlook at Tulane as far as building up a department is concerned is absolutely hopeless. The university is dependent upon Charity Hospital, a state institution that is in the control

---

106 Salvaggio, *New Orleans' Charity Hospital.*
107 Ibid.

of politics. The university is merely tolerated in the hospital and there is no cooperation at all."[108] After placing a copy of the letter in his coat, Ochsner later found the letter missing. Not long after, someone presented the letter to Governor Huey P. Long and the hospital board, which resulted in the termination of Ochsner's appointment to the hospital's visiting staff.

After this event, Tulane then refused to grant Long the honorary doctor of law degree that he desired. Long did not hide his animosity toward Tulane, and three months after Ochsner's dismissal it was announced that Louisiana State University would have its own medical school that would open in 1931. Governor Long stated, "Honest boys with good records come out of LSU and can't get into that medical school… We're a-going to fix that."[109] In order to raise the considerable funds for a medical school, Long had LSU illegally sell land to the state for a new capitol building and highway commission. By the time he was taken to court for the nearly $2.15 million in state bonds spent, the school was already built and "the court had to shrug its shoulders."[110] In 1931 the LSU School of Medicine opened on the grounds of the Charity complex along Tulane Avenue. Arthur Vidrine, the personal physician of Long, headed the school; he had previously been rebuffed by Tulane when he sought a professorship in surgery and later a professorship in head and neck surgery. He had had training in neither.[111]

Dr. Urban Maes, a well-respected New Orleans private practice surgeon, eventually headed the LSU surgery department. This appointment would give the school much-needed credibility. Maes only accepted the position under the condition that Ochsner be reinstated to Charity; this would be the

---

108 Ibid.
109 Ibid.
110 Ibid.
111 Ibid.

beginning of easing tensions between the LSU and Tulane surgery departments.[112]

However, political embroilments with Long did not change. At the time, doctors treated wealthy Long supporters for free at Charity, and 5 percent was deducted from all hospital salaries to support Long's campaign funds. The entire hospital atmosphere was "one of fear of Long's possible reprisals if one did not do what he or his henchman wanted...It was, in essence, a police state."[113]

However, on September 10, 1935, Long was assassinated, and Vidrine quickly lost his post as the head of the school. Long left Charity in dire financial straits after his death. While a senator, to discredit his political enemy President Franklin Roosevelt, Long had spearheaded a law stating that Louisiana would not take any federal money to fund operations such as Charity Hospital, leaving it with little source of income after his death. It is local lore that immediately after he was shot, Long asked to be treated by Ochsner. However, Ochsner still felt bitter about their relationship and outright refused. Thus Vidrine operated on Long with the aid of Baton Rouge surgeons but was unable to save his life.[114]

Ochsner's era not only heralded advances in medical education, but also in adding surgical specialties to the department's repertoire. In 1934, Tulane University established a plastic surgery program when Neal Owens became the first instructor of plastic surgery. Having trained at the University of Alabama and Emory University, Owens received a commission to work in London in 1933 with Sir Harold Gillies—the father of plastic and facial reconstructive surgery.[115] Returning at the end of that year with little money, Owens wrote to ten professors of surgery regarding their interest in developing plastic surgery at their

112 Ibid.
113 Ibid.
114 Ibid.
115 Richard Hollingham, *Blood and Guts: A History of Surgery* (Great Britain: Edbury Publishing, 2008).

institutions. Of the three that replied, only Dr. Alton Ochsner at Tulane replied with an affirmative interest. However, during his interview with Owens, Dr. Ochsner painted "the blackest picture about possibilities,"[116] and, in fact, Owens was initially appointed with no salary. Owens and Ochsner would go on to work together on many cases, including one to construct a substitute esophagus for a little girl whose natural esophagus had been closed due to drinking lye.[117]

During his tenure, Dr. Owens developed the first plastic surgery training program in New Orleans. Working mainly at Charity Hospital, he was also chief of plastic surgery at the Eye, Ear, Nose, and Throat Hospital and an attending surgeon at Touro Infirmary, Hotel Dieu, and Mercy and Sara Mayo Hospitals. Much of his service was to victims of head, neck, and skin cancer, and he contributed greatly to the development of treatments for burn victims, as well as cleft lip and palate patients. Following the development of the Crippled Children's Program in Louisiana, Dr. Owens performed about twenty such surgeries per month. Apart from his own surgical accomplishments, Dr. Owens trained over thirty plastic surgeons, many of whom became leaders in the field. The plastic surgery residency program was officially established in 1968. The first residents of the program were Hans M. Tschopp and Gustavo Colon.[118] The program is currently comprised of five years of general surgery and three years of plastic surgery residency.

The establishment of the New Orleans clinic that bore Ochsner's name was exceedingly controversial and in many ways was based on restrictions for Tulane staff at Charity and Tulane University's lack of its own hospital. Ochsner had pushed for Tulane to create its own university hospital even before World War II; however, he was met with much concern that it would "damage the university's academic reputation." In 1941, Och-

---

116 "Arthur Neal Owens, M.D. (1899–1985)." *Plastic & Reconstructive Surgery* 77, no. 2 (February 1986): 353–55.
117 Wilds and Harkey, *Alton Ochsner: Surgeon of the South*, p. 118–119.
118 Interview with Gustavo Colon, August 15, 2010.

sner, along with four colleagues at Tulane, founded the Ochsner Clinic. Ochsner's colleagues were Edgar Burns (urology), Guy Caldwell (orthopedics), Francis LeJeune (ear, nose, and throat), and Curtis Tyrone (ob/gyn). The five Tulane affiliated surgeons staffed it, and it initially opened next to the Touro Infirmary. However, it soon moved to Camp Plauche military hospital in 1947 and then to its current site in 1954. Although envisioned as a potential partner institution with Tulane, the university's board of administrators, the medical school, and the New Orleans medical community did not welcome the new clinic.[119] In fact, on "Holy Thursday" night, April 13, 1941, in an obvious reference to Judas Iscariot, each of the founders received a leather sack containing thirty dimes, with a note: "To help pay for your Clinic. From the Physicians, Surgeons, and Dentists of New Orleans."[120] Although initial relations were obviously strained, Tulane and the Ochsner Clinic would later collaborate in a variety of areas throughout the years.

One of Ochsner's most famous students was Michael DeBakey, one of the pioneers of cardiothoracic surgery. While Ochsner was known for being understanding and mild mannered, the residents referred to DeBakey as "Black Mike" for his hard-nosed attitude and poor bedside matter.[121]

Michael E. DeBakey was born in Lake Charles, Louisiana, on September 7, 1908. He was born into a very wealthy but strict family. His parents prioritized reading and studying. In fact, DeBakey had read the entire *Encyclopedia Britannica* before going to college.[122] DeBakey earned his bachelor's degree from Tulane University while enrolling in the medical school at the same time; he was the first to earn a degree from both in 1932. While doing research in a physics lab as an undergrad, DeBakey first got his idea for the roller pump, which would change the face of surgery twenty years later as the heart-lung machine,

---

119 Haslam, *Dr. Mary's Monkey.*
120 Ibid., p. 145.
121 Salvaggio, *New Orleans' Charity Hospital.*
122 *DeBakey: A Documentary Film* (video, screening copy), June 22, 2011.

making open heart surgery a possibility. While still an under-grad student at Tulane, he used his primitive roller pump for blood transfusions and was requested by doctors all over town to assist with transfusions.[123] After completing his residency at Charity Hospital, he went to the University of Strasbourg in France at the urging of Dr. Matas and the University of Heidelberg in Germany at the urging of Dr. Ochsner, returning to the United States before World War II. After this, he returned to Tulane, serving on the surgery faculty from 1937 to 1948, earning three thousand dollars a year.[124] Staff members described him as "an extraordinary man and superb surgical technician who would perform a complex surgical procedure and make it look simple, yet he would rarely see a patient after an operation."[125]

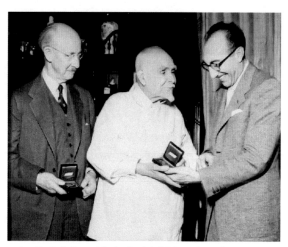

Dr. Matas presenting Dr. Debakey with the Rudolph Matas Award in Vascular Surgery in 1954.

He took leave during World War II to work for the United States Surgeon General, trying to improve the medical condition of soldiers while in the field. He worked on preventing

123 William Roberts, "Michael Ellis DeBakey: A Conversation with the Editor." *Am J of Cardiology* 79 (1997): 929–50.
124 Roberts, "Michael Ellis DeBakey."
125 Salvaggio, *New Orleans' Charity Hospital.*

hypothermia as well as developing Mobile Army Surgical Hospital (MASH) units, developments that decreased wounded mortality to 4.4 percent—an unprecedented low.[126] After the war, thousands of wounded soldiers came back to the United States. The government asked DeBakey to stay in service an extra year and work with a team of over one hundred surgeons to reorganize the Veterans Administration (VA) system to take care of these soldiers. He brought the hospitals from all the branches of the military under the VA system and also tried to link the major VA hospitals to medical schools. In 1948, he was offered the chair of a young surgery department at Baylor University in Houston. He transformed Baylor into the medical institution that it is today. He also helped develop the VA system there, integrating it into the university.[127]

DeBakey also used his fame and medical expertise in the political arena as well. He worked to form the National Library of Medicine—Medline is a branch of this that is commonly used today.[128] He was a member of the Hoover Commission that developed health care policy, and he served as council to many US presidents. He was the personal surgeon of most sitting US presidents, Prince Edward, King Leopold, Marshal Tito (president of Yugoslavia), the shah of Iran, Boris Yeltsin, Frank Sinatra, and many other celebrities. He also had many firsts accredited to his name:[129] first to perform coronary artery bypass surgery, perform carotid endarterectomy, use Dacron grafts, perform angioplasty with patch grafts, use cardiac assist device, and many more. He also created a left ventricular assist device that is widely used today. DeBakey continued to practice medicine until his death, at nearly one hundred years of age.

Many have asked why DeBakey left Tulane and why he did not return after Ochsner left. In an interview, DeBakey stated that he left because he and Ochsner were the same age and he

---

126 *DeBakey: A Documentary Film.*
127 Ibid.
128 Ibid.
129 Ibid.

did not want the competition to interfere with their friendship. He saw an opportunity in Houston and seized it. After Ochsner left Tulane, DeBakey felt that the fledgling Baylor University was too dependent on him and that he needed to stay and continue to support it.[130]

Like many men who obtain a multitude of great achievements, Ochsner was not without controversy—even to this day. In 2007 Edward Haslam published a book entitled *Dr. Mary's Monkey*. It alleges that Ochsner was a prominent member of the Information Council of the Americas (INCA) and had an internationalist view that may have helped secure secret government contracts for cancer viral research. Ochsner was known for being very involved in politics and extremely well connected in New Orleans and across the United States. The fact that he is still a topic of conversation on the international stage nearly a century later speaks volumes for the accomplishments of a boy who grew up in rural South Dakota.

After thirty years of service to the Department of Surgery, Dr. Ochsner resigned as chair of the Department of Surgery, although he maintained his position as clinical professor of surgery.

---

130 Roberts, "Michael Ellis DeBakey."

Oscar Creech Jr., 1956–1967

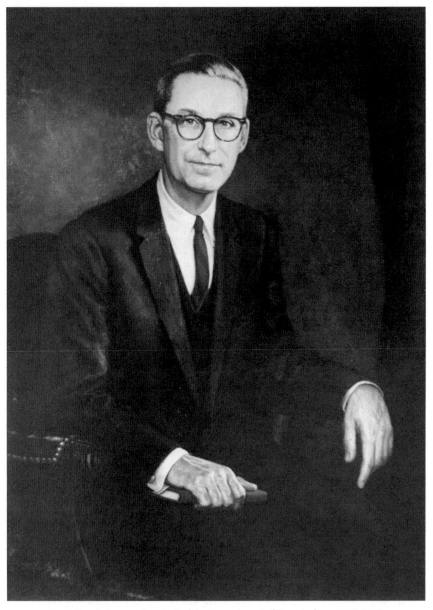

Oscar Creech Jr. served as chair of the Department of Surgery from 1956–1967.

Dr. Oscar Creech succeeded Ochsner in 1956. Creech had received his medical degree from Jefferson Medical College in Philadelphia prior to completing his residency in surgery under Dr. Ochsner at Tulane. When his Tulane mentor, Michael DeBakey, accepted the chairmanship of surgery at Baylor Medical College in 1949, Creech followed and joined the faculty there where they further improved upon the Dacron vascular graft. He returned to New Orleans and Tulane in 1956 to assume the chairmanship of surgery. Dr. Creech served for eleven years until he accepted the position of dean of the medical school in July 1967. He passed away from lymphoma in December of that year.

Dr. Creech was one of the few physicians to receive two Hektoen medals from the American Medical Association. One was for his work with Michael DeBakey on aortic replacement, and the other was for his work with Edward Krementz and Robert Ryan on regional perfusion.[131] The 1950s saw the groundbreaking work by Edward Krementz, Oscar Creech, and Robert Ryan at Tulane in the development of the regional perfusion technique, which allowed for concentration of chemotherapeutic agents into isolated regions of the body using the heart-lung pumps without increasing toxicity in other portions of the body. This was found to be beneficial in cases of malignant melanoma, pelvic cancers, carcinomas, and soft tissue sarcomas.[132] This development was awarded the Hektoen medal in 1959 and is still used today. Years later, Dr. Ryan related the story that the collaboration actually started at a cocktail party in February 1957, during which Drs. Creech and Krementz lamented the status of cancer treatment in the New Orleans area.[133]

---

131 Robert F. Ryan, *One of the Golden Ages of Tulane Surgery* (New Orleans, LA: Robert F. Ryan, 2006), p. 8.

132 "Historic Study of Perfusion." *Medical World News*, August 17, 1962, p. 28–30.

133 Edward T. Krementz, R. Davilene Carter, Carl M. Sutherland, James H. Muchmore, Robert F. Ryan, and Oscar Creech Jr., "Regional Chemotherapy for Melanoma: A 35-Year Experience." *Annals of Surgery* 220, no. 4 (October 1994): 520–35.

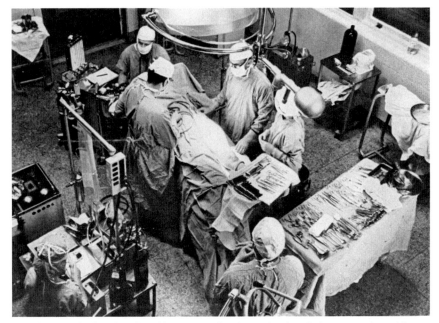

Photograph of Dr. Creech and his team performing regional perfusion on a patient with malignant melanoma of the leg.

Dr. Oscar Creech recruited Dr. Krementz from Yale University; Krementz served as head of the surgical oncology section, as well as the director of the Tulane Cancer Clinical Research Center from 1961 to 1975. According to Dr. Robert Ryan, Dr. Krementz was the first physician to give chemotherapy (nitrogen mustard) for a malignancy when he applied it to a malignant melanoma that had been grown in the eye of a guinea pig.[134] Dr. Krementz retired in 1989 after more than forty years of service to the department and many advances in the world of surgical oncology.

Dr. Creech's had a well-deserved reputation as a leader in cardiovascular surgery, and he earned citations from the American Heart Association during his career. He performed

134 Ryan, *One of the Golden Ages of Tulane Surgery*, p. 10.

the first open-heart operation in New Orleans with use of the extracorporeal pump.

Apart from his surgical skills, Dr. Creech was a respected administrator and teacher. He held a surgical clinic for students, residents, and faculty on a weekly basis. Also, he was the first to appoint a professor of scientific communications in order to teach both students and doctors at the medical school how to present scientific material in a clear and understandable manner. His lectures were always well attended and spiced with humor.[135] To this day, surgeons look back and remember him as a kind and gentle educator who garnered the respect of all of those around him. Those who were part of his team were always very hard working, not out of fear, but out of a desire not to disappoint Dr. Creech.[136]

There are many anecdotes of the character of Dr. Creech. In the 1950s, Dr. Claude Organ (who would go on to become the second African American president of the American College of Surgeons) visited Tulane. At that time, the restaurants of New Orleans were not integrated. Instead of having Dr. Organ suffer the embarrassment of having to enter the restaurant through a side door, Dr. Creech paid for a chef to come to Dr. Ryan's house, and they all had dinner there on Dr. Creech's dime.[137]

Dr. Creech's 1963 Ivy Day speech, which presented a forceful and documented call for the establishment of a university hospital by Tulane University, was instrumental in the establishment of Tulane University Hospital. In his speech, he declared that as a result of years of political patronage, Charity's nursing staff had been depleted, its clinical laboratories performed only the simplest procedures, its x-ray department had seriously curtailed services, and some of the operating rooms had been closed. "The truth of the matter is, it is impossible to teach or to learn medicine here as it should be practiced and

135 Letter from Philip Brewer, June 28, 2011.
136 Interview with James Brown, November 15, 2012.
137 Ryan, *One of the Golden Ages of Tulane Surgery*, p. 10.

as it is being practiced in other teaching hospitals."[138] To get an idea of the state of Charity in the 1960s, reports state that on an average day there were 10,000 people (patients, visitors, employees, etc.) in the facility, with 500,000 patients seen each year; it was the world's largest outpatient center, it delivered 6,000 babies each year, and it answered 22,000 ambulance calls. It did all this on $33.9 million per year. To put this in perspective, comparable Cook County Hospital worked on $65 million and LA County on $100 million per year budgets.[139]

There are many stories that describe life in Charity Hospital at that time. In one, a ward nurse who had an invalid child could not afford to raise him at home, so he stayed on the ward that she worked on for nearly thirteen years. Charity doctors often treated prisoners from Angola Prison. The smart prisoners would develop "conditions requiring a long stay," with the residents teaching them to record vitals and ins-and-outs on patients. If prison officials ever inquired about the prisoners, they would "quickly recover" and be sent back to the prison.[140] In another story, an elderly nun would come to the emergency department for care of her venous ulcers. Over eighteen "complete" history and physicals were documented on her over two years only for a staff physician to discover that the nun was actually a man on his nineteenth visit.[141]

In 1969, the administrators of the Tulane Educational Fund established the Tulane Medical Center in order to implement the medical school's plans for expansion. To guide this process, they established a Board of Governors with the authority to implement those plans. The Tulane University Hospital and Clinic was the first university teaching hospital in Louisiana. Groundbreaking ceremonies were held on December 1, 1973, and the official dedication was held on September 23, 1976. Located across from the medical school on Tulane Avenue, the

---

138 Duffy, *The Tulane University Medical Center.*
139 Salvaggio, *New Orleans' Charity Hospital.*
140 Interview with James Brown, November 15, 2012.
141 Salvaggio, *New Orleans' Charity Hospital.*

three-hundred-bed hospital provided not only a wide range of patient services, but also greatly expanded Tulane's ability to offer clinical instruction for its students and research opportunities for its faculty.[142]

During his tenure as chair of the Department of Surgery, Dr. Creech oversaw an increase of grant money from the National Institutes of Health (NIH) awarded to the Tulane School of Medicine. In fact, his laundry budget for the laboratory during his first year as chair was larger than Dr. Ochsner's entire research budget at its greatest.[143]

Dr. Creech also established Tulane's transplant program with the selection of Dr. Keith Reemtsma to lead the department's efforts. Dr. Reemtsma joined the faculty during the 1957–1958 academic year following receipt of his medical degrees from the University of Pennsylvania and Columbia University. His training at Columbia was interrupted by his military service during the Korean War. According to his wife, Reemtsma's military service became the model for the character Dr. Hawkeye Pierce in the film and television series *M*A*S*H*.[144]

Dr. Reemtsma's work in the field of xenotransplantation while at Tulane established his reputation as a pioneer in transplantation surgery. On November 4, 1963, Reemtsma transplanted kidneys from a chimpanzee into a forty-three-year old man suffering from kidney and heart failure at Tulane. The patient lived eight weeks. In all, Reemtsma performed a dozen chimpanzee-to-human kidney transplants during 1963 and 1964, with one patient, a twenty-three-year old woman, surviving nine months with no sign of rejection.[145] Tissue typing was rudimentary in the 1960s, with the patients dying of overwhelming infections from immunosuppression or by fatal "graft vs. host" reactions. In addition, patients with monkey kidneys had complications from low

142 Duffy, *The Tulane University Medical Center.*
143 Interview with Robert L. Hewitt, July 6, 2010.
144 Lawrence Altma, "Keith Reemtsma, 74, Pioneer in Medical Transplants, Dies." *New York Times* (June 28, 2000).
145 Salvaggio, *New Orleans' Charity Hospital.*

potassium.[146] It was soon learned that normal potassium levels in a monkey were too low to be compatible with life for humans. Thus, monkey transplantation was abandoned. While such surgeries were controversial, Reemtsma believed "it's important to realize this started at a time when it was a medical necessity" because kidney dialysis and transplants from human cadavers were unavailable at the time.[147] Tulane would eventually begin transplanting human kidneys and, in a venture with Charity, opened a ten-bed transplant unit in 1966. Reemtsma would continue to work on transplantation, starting research on transplantation of pancreatic islet cells for treatment of diabetes.[148]

Dr. John C. McDonald was another pioneer in the area of transplantation surgery at Tulane. Dr. McDonald received his medical degree from Tulane in 1955 and served as professor of surgery and head of the transplantation section at the State University of New York–Buffalo before returning to Tulane in 1968. During that year, he was appointed associate professor of microbiology and immunology and was named the director of the transplantation laboratory.

Dr. McDonald considered the production of acquired immunologic tolerance in humans to be the Holy Grail of transplantation surgery. His research in this area focused on the importance of cellular and humoral immunity, transplant rejection, and the development of methods to detect early rejection episodes. Along with a team of kidney transplant specialists, Dr. McDonald discovered a system that was found to be responsible for acute transplantation rejection, which they called the Heterophile Transplantation Antigen,

---

146 Ibid.
147 "Organs of Species" (newspaper article, undated), Department of Surgery PR files, Rudolph Matas Library.
148 John C. McDonald, M.D., "These Are Surgeons at Tulane," http://johncmcdonald.org/pop-html/article0069.html (accessed April 9, 2012).

or HTA, System.[149] McDonald left Tulane in 1977 to become chair of the surgery department at LSU in Shreveport.[150]

The department also recruited Dr. Ambrose Storck during this era. He was known for his immense surgical ability and for being the most eligible bachelor in New Orleans, often seen driving down Canal Street in his Packard car and wearing fine white linen suits. He had a thriving private practice but would spend time with the residents doing cases in the animal lab and at Charity, always elaborating on the finer points of the surgical procedures. Even senior residents and other staff would walk away from cases with a sense of awe.[151]

Edward Thomas Krementz, 1967–1968 (Acting)

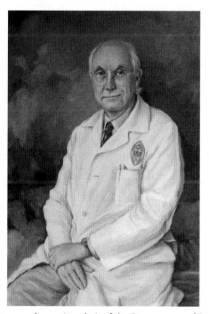

Edward Tomas Krementz served as acting chair of the Department of Surgery from 1967–1968.

149 John C. McDonald, M.D., "Transplantation Contributions," http://johncmcdonald.org/transplantation.html (Accessed July 15, 2010).
150 John C. McDonald, M.D., "These Are Surgeons at Tulane."
151 Ryan, *One of the Golden Ages of Tulane Surgery.*

Following Dr. Creech's appointment as dean of the medical school in 1967, his colleague and co-inventor of the regional perfusion technique, Dr. Edward Krementz, served as acting chairman of the Department of Surgery until Theodore Drapanas assumed the position on September 1, 1968.

Theodore Drapanas, 1968–1975

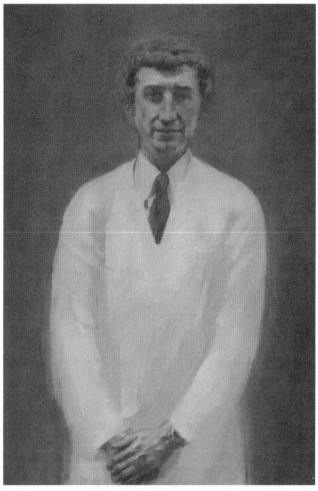

Theodore Drapanas served as chair of the Department of Surgery from 1968–1975.

Dr. Drapanas was only the second chair of the Tulane Department of Surgery who had not received his medical training from the university since the residency program started. Nonetheless, he brought with him a solid reputation as a surgeon. Dr. Drapanas received his MD from the University of Buffalo and taught at the University of Pittsburgh Medical School from 1964–1968.

Dr. Drapanas continued the tradition of excellence in teaching and was selected the Outstanding Educator of the Year in the School of Medicine in 1970. Dr. Drapanas was also an innovative surgeon. He worked to develop the interposition mesocaval shunt as a treatment for portal hypertension using a Dacron graft anastomosed between the inferior vena cava and the superior mesenteric vein, which became known as a "Drapanas shunt."

During his tenure as chairman, he and Dr. John McDonald led Tulane's transplantation program to national prominence and performed the first liver transplant in Louisiana in 1972.[152]

Drapanas had varied research interests. These included liver transplant studies, analyses of critically ill patients, the mechanism of pulmonary failure during shock, and notably surgical corrections of portal hypertension through the use of shunts. He published over eighty articles and books throughout his career.

Drapanas was well-read and published many manuscripts. In one event, he and Dr. Nance, from the LSU surgery department, studied that exact same patient population at Charity and drew opposite conclusions on how to deal with pancreatic trauma at the time. They would go on to present their data and debate their opinions publicly at a national conference. To prevent another embarrassing moment like this in the future, administrators quickly put a system into place so that Tulane and LSU would have to sign off on publications by the other

---

152 John C. McDonald, MD, "Transplantation Contributions."

department when either manuscript was examining Charity patients.[153]

Drapanas oversaw a large surgical department that had boomed under the era of Dr. Creech. He had a budget of slightly over eight hundred thousand dollars to run the general surgery, orthopedics, neurosurgery, and urology departments.[154]

A plane crash June 1975 at John F. Kennedy International Airport tragically cut short Dr. Drapanas's life and tenure as chair. At the time of his death, he was a member of numerous medical organizations and the editor of *Surgery*, which carried a tribute to him in its September 1975 issue. He was still very young in his career, and many felt that he was on the verge of many groundbreaking discoveries in the field of transplantation and surgery as a whole.[155]

Robert Frank Ryan, 1975–1977 (Acting)

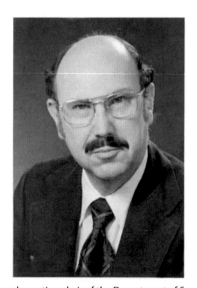

Robert Frank Ryan served as acting chair of the Department of Surgery from 1975–1977.

153 Interview with Norman McSwain, November 16, 2012.
154 "Tulane Surgery Department Quarterly Budget Review," July 1, 1973, to June 30, 1974.
155 Duffy, *The Tulane University Medical Center.*

Dr. Robert Frank Ryan served as acting chairman during the search for Dr. Drapanas's replacement. In addition to his previously mentioned medical achievements, Dr. Ryan was known for his investments, both in business and in people. One notable investment was in the now-famous Louisiana folk artist Clementine Hunter.[156] Clementine Hunter was born on the Hidden Hill Plantation (said to be the inspiration for *Uncle Tom's Cabin*) in Natchitoches Parish, Louisiana, around 1887— the exact date is unknown. At the age of fifteen, she moved to Melrose Plantation, where she worked most of her life as a field hand. Melrose Plantation had become a popular retreat for artists at that time, and, at the age of fifty, Clementine Hunter taught herself to paint using discarded brushes and oil paints. She painted on anything she could get a hold of, including cardboard boxes, gourds, and lampshades.[157] In the 1960s, Dr. Ryan began making monthly trips to the Charity Hospital in Alexandria, Louisiana. On one such trip, he met Clementine. He was immediately drawn to her work because, "unlike the depressing modern art of the era, [Clementine's art] was bright, cheerful, and not morbid."[158]

It took nearly a year before Clementine would warm up to Dr. Ryan. Over their twenty-seven-year relationship, Dr. Ryan acquired roughly seven hundred pieces of her art, which would become the largest private collection of her work. He would sometimes pay her ten to two hundred dollars per piece, or simply trade her for supplies, such as paints and toothpaste. Dr. Ryan even had an influence on her work. He would bring pictures of Clementine and have her incorporate them into her paintings.[159] Near the end of her life, when her hands were becoming stiff with arthritis, he would

---

156 Interview with Ronald Nichols, November 13, 2012.
157 Landscape Online, "Melrose Plantation," http://www.landscapeonline.com/research (accessed February 14, 2013).
158 Doug MacCash, "Hunter Gatherer," *NOLA*, July 27, 2007.
159 Southern Visionary Art, "Clementine Hunter," http://www.southernvisionaryart.com/gallery-clementinehunter (accessed February 14, 2013).

glue small canvases to tongue depressors for her so she could paint easier. Now, those ten dollar pieces of art depicting daily life on a Louisiana plantation are worth thousands of dollars. Today, much of Dr. Ryan's collection can be seen at the Ogden Museum of Southern Art.[160]

Watts Webb, 1977–1989

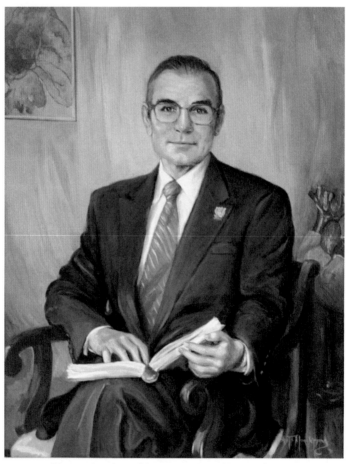

Watts Webb served as chair of the Department of Surgery from 1977–1989.

---

160 MacCash, "Hunter Gatherer."

After a two-year search, Dr. Watts R. Webb joined the Tulane faculty as chairman of the department on May 1, 1977. Trained at the University of Mississippi and Barnes Hospital in St. Louis, Dr. Webb brought with him experience as a leader in cardio-thoracic surgery and as a departmental chair. Prior to joining the faculty at Tulane, Dr. Webb had served as chairman of the Thoracic and Cardiovascular Surgery Division at the University of Texas Southwestern Medical School and chairman of surgery at the Upstate Medical Center at SUNY–Syracuse.

Webb was well-known as a "Southern Surgeon" through and through. He came from a very strict residency program where residents were not allowed to get married or have long hair. While he was not this dictatorial, he was very stern and strict with the surgery department. Under his organization and leadership, the department would grow and flourish. Webb would remain chairman of the department until Tulane's mandatory retirement age of sixty-five. At that time, he went on to become chairman at LSU.[161]

Webb, upon coming to New Orleans, soon recruited Dr. Norman McSwain and Dr. Ronald Nichols, who would both make great advances for the program. They arrived on nearly the same day in 1977 and continue to work with the program to this day.

---

161 Interview with Norman McSwain, November 16, 2012.

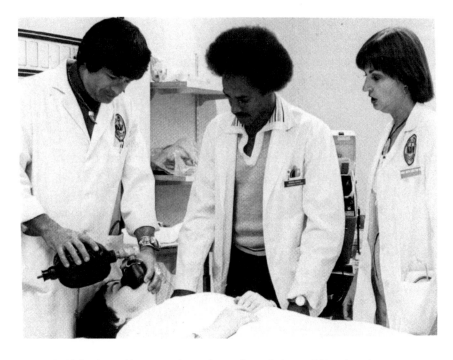

Dr. McSwain teaching proper bag-valve mask ventilation to EMT students in 1978.

In 1977, Dr. Norman McSwain joined the staff of the Department of Surgery to work at Charity Hospital and establish an Emergency Medical System (EMS) in New Orleans. During the mid-1970s, ambulance services were provided by five to six companies in New Orleans, and service was erratic at times. Some nights all six services were operating, and other nights no services would be operating.[162] The first Charity Hospital ambulance service began in 1885 and was staffed by the interns for nearly one hundred years. On its first run, it had taken the ambulance so long to arrive that the patient had already recovered and left the scene. Not wanting to return empty handed, the intern grabbed "an unsuspecting negro and brought him

---

162 Interview with Norman McSwain, November 16, 2012.

back to the hospital."[163] By the time Dr. McSwain arrived, interns were no longer running the ambulance services.

Dr. McSwain studied medicine at the University of Alabama's School of Medicine and the Bowman-Gray School of Medicine in Winston-Salem, North Carolina, before receiving additional training in the US Air Force and at the Grady Memorial Hospital in Atlanta. He joined the medical staff at the University of Kansas and established the EMS system for the state of Kansas.

The reputation of Charity Hospital as a prominent trauma center attracted Dr. McSwain to join the faculty at Tulane. After coming to Tulane, he initiated a citywide EMS system and the EMT-Basic and EMT-Paramedic training within the New Orleans Police Department (NOPD). Early in his career at Tulane, Dr. McSwain also began serving as the police surgeon for the NOPD.[164]

In 1975 the American Heart Association provided Advanced Cardiac Life Support (ACLS) training. Dr. McSwain was sent to the course and, after completion, felt that a similar course was needed for trauma surgery. He took this idea to the American College of Surgeons and was the ad hoc chair for the establishment of the Advanced Trauma Life Support (ATLS) course. The course provides orientation in the "initial assessment and management of the trauma victim by a series of lectures and practical stations." After they created the course in Lincoln, Nebraska, they began distributing it to each region in the United States. In 1978, Dr. McSwain began ATLS education at Tulane for its surgery residents. He also began using a version for the paramedic program (which was started in late 1977) to train the EMTs in New Orleans to the paramedic level. After three years, the state of Louisiana moved the paramedic training program to Charity Hospital.[165] Mary Beth Skelton and Joe Nigliazzo took over the running of the ATLS and ACLS programs for the department.

163 Salvaggio, *New Orleans' Charity Hospital.*
164 Interview with Norman McSwain, November 16, 2012.
165 Interview with Norman McSwain, November 15, 2012.

Later, Peggy Chehardy ran the programs at the School of Medicine. From 2006 to 2008, Dr. Chehardy served as director of the Tulane Trauma Educational Institute, which provides annual ATLS courses for physicians, as well as nurses, paramedics, and other allied health professionals.[166]

Dr. Ronald Nichols received his medical degree from the University of Illinois Medical School and a master of science in surgery degree from the University of Illinois Graduate School. After completing residency in surgery, he became faculty at the University of Illinois Medical Center and shortly thereafter became faculty at Chicago Medical School. He was recruited by Dr. Webb at a Central Surgical Meeting and was offered an endowed surgical chair and a research lab. With this offer, Dr. Nichols moved his family to New Orleans.[167]

---

166 Tulane University, "Advanced Trauma Life Support Course Description," http://tulane.edu/ som/departments/surgery/ home/upload/2010.pdf (accessed October 20, 2010).

167 Interview with Ronald Nichols, November 13, 2012.

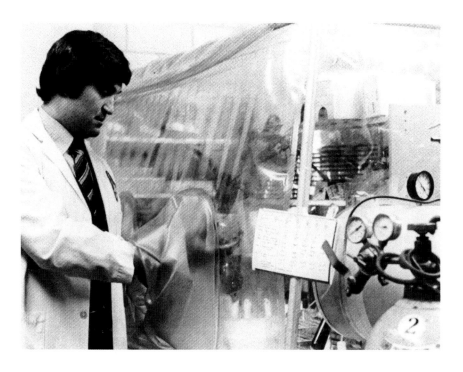

Dr. Nichols working with an anaerobic bacteria chamber in 1978.

One of Dr. Nichols's greatest contributions to the world of surgery and infectious disease was the creation of the Nichols-Condon Bowel Prep. He began thinking about surgical wounds while in residency and noticed that patients with intestinal and colon surgery had more wound infections and that the dressings smelled fouler than the others. He would routinely send the purulence to the microbiology lab, but they were never able to grow anything. Seeing organisms on the gram stain, he knew that they were missing something. The advent of anaerobic cultures a few years later would greatly change our understanding of the bowel flora.[168]

Now being able to culture anaerobes, Dr. Nichols did a set of experiments defining the microbial flora of the bowel. Dur-

168 Interview with Ronald Nichols, November 13, 2012.

ing surgical procedures, he would aspirate the contents of the terminal ileum, cecum, and transverse colon. He published his flora results, then linked these results to the high infection rates in GI cases. He used this data to develop the neomycin/erythromycin bowel prep that is still used to this day.[169]

The Infectious Diseases Society of America accepted Dr. Nichols as one of the only non-internal medicine physicians, and Tulane made him a professor of microbiology. He had a robust research lab operating in the medical school from 1977 to 2000. He would continue on to define infection rates and risk in penetrating abdominal patients, publish over 180 articles, and write 130 book chapters. He is now an emeritus professor for the Department of Surgery.[170]

The opening of the Tulane University Hospital in 1976 was an important factor in Dr. Webb's decision to join the Tulane faculty.[171] The development of the university hospital allowed Tulane to expand its clinical opportunities for students and residents, as well as provide increased research capabilities for faculty.

By the mid-twentieth century, Tulane placed further emphasis on student involvement in clinical work and in informal conferences while keeping to a minimum hours devoted to formal lectures in the surgery department. First-year students were introduced to terminology and fundamental concepts of surgery, while students were taught physical examination, diagnosis, and emergency management of certain acute conditions during the second year. Juniors within the medical school spent twelve weeks in the Department of Surgery during which they engaged in clinical clerkships at Charity Hospital and outpatient clinics. Instruction during the final year included a focus on surgical specialties, as well as surgical care of patients, with students assigned to Charity or Touro Infir-

169 Interview with Ronald Nichols, November 13, 2012.
170 Interview with Ronald Nichols, November 13, 2012.
171 Interview with Watts Webb, August 2, 2010.

mary and as externs to Huey P. Long Charity Hospital and Lallie Kemp Charity Hospital.

During the decade of the 1960s, instruction in surgery at Tulane changed in order to mirror the growth of specialization within the surgical field (and in medicine as a whole). Prior to 1964, courses within the department had focused on general surgery, orthopedic surgery, otolaryngology, and urology, with instruction in disaster medicine, pathology, surgical physiology, plastic surgery, and neurological surgery also provided. In 1965, Tulane added a tumor conference for juniors and seniors as part of the general surgery course. The following year introduced clinics in proctology, vascular surgery, and thoracic surgery, and a thoracic and cardiovascular conference was offered beginning in 1967. Electives that year included emergency surgery and trauma, as well as oncology, and a seminar on plastic surgery. By the end of the decade, electives included courses on cardiovascular surgery, transplantation surgery, cancer research, pediatric electrocardiography, and proctology.

Apart from surgical training, Tulane developed and offered an elective in scientific communication beginning in the early 1960s, marking the first time a curriculum-approved communication course was offered in a medical school.[172] The course for undergraduate students was "designed to improve competence in use of the English language and to provide incentive for continued improvement in writing and speech by application of the principles of effective self-expression."[173] The course was taught by Lois DeBakey; her brother and former Tulane surgical professor Michael DeBakey had suggested the course as a way of teaching doctors to communicate more

---

172 An article by Ronda Wendler entitled "DeBakey Sisters Teach Logic and Language of Medicine" on the Texas Medical Center website (http://www.texasmedicalcenter.org/root/en/TMCServices/News/2008/05-01/DeBakey+Sisters.htm) states the course was initially taught in 1962, but it did not appear in the Tulane School of Medicine catalogue until the 1965/1966 academic year (accessed July 5, 2010).
173 Tulane University School of Medicine, *Bulletin, 1965–1966.*, p. 85.

effectively and plainly with patients—in other words, to speak less "medicalese."

The establishment of Tulane University Hospital in 1976 allowed the university to expand its clinical instruction at both the undergraduate and postgraduate levels. Clerkships in the undergraduate program expanded into a wider array of specialty areas.

With a strong general surgery residency already in place, residencies included the areas of cardiothoracic surgery, vascular surgery, and plastic surgery, as well as fellowships in oncology, trauma, and vascular surgery.

Growth in faculty from the late 1970s to the late 1980s expanded the department's divisions, as well. Patricia C. Moynihan joined the faculty with a dual appointment in pediatrics and surgery. Jack Hussey reactivated the transplantation program with a particular focus on renal and pancreatic transplants. Norman McSwain's recruitment and his experience in the management of trauma led to Tulane's leadership in the area of trauma and critical care. The addition of Morris Kerstein strengthened Tulane's work in the area of vascular surgery.

While the opening of the Louisiana State University Medical Center in 1931 and the Ochsner Clinic in 1941 had provided competition for surgical training in New Orleans, the growth of those institutions also pushed Tulane to continually expand and focus its work on surgical research, teaching, and clinic care throughout the decades. By the late 1980s, New Orleans was indeed a very competitive environment for surgery, particularly with the growth of the LSU School of Medicine and its associations with Charity Hospital and the local VA Hospital.

Lewis M. Flint, 1989–1999

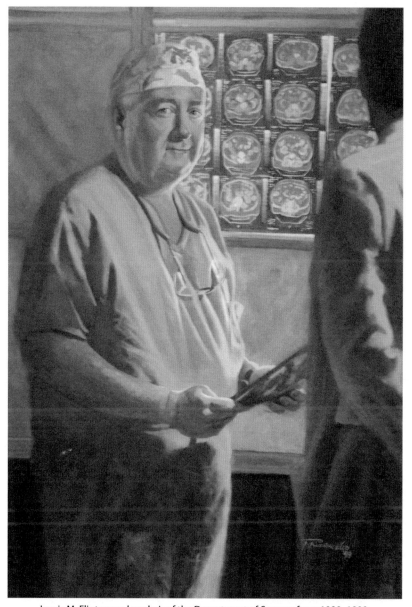

Lewis M. Flint served as chair of the Department of Surgery from 1989–1999.

It was this environment that met Dr. Lewis Flint when he assumed the chair of the Department of Surgery in 1989 following Dr. Webb's departure to the LSU faculty.[174]

Dr. Flint went to medical school and did his residency at Duke University. He was practicing in New York when he was recruited to come to Tulane. Dr. Flint was known to be quiet and introverted, but he was given a lot of support from the medical school to expand the department. Dr. Flint had a photographic memory and could often rattle off page numbers and citations of medical literature during residents' morbidity and mortality conferences.[175]

During Dr. Flint's years as chair, the Department of Surgery focused on excellence in education, research, and clinical care. The latter proved to be particularly challenging due to competing clinical care facilities at Ochsner and LSU, but during this time, Tulane responded to such challenges by developing its congenital heart disease program and its multiorgan transplant program. Dr. Flint recruited Drs. Douglas Slakey and Stephen Cheng to assist in the development of the transplant program and Dr. Donald Akers to lead the division of vascular surgery. While faculty such as Drs. Slakey and Akers led specialty areas, from an education standpoint, the department focused on general surgery during the Flint years in order to provide its students and residents training in the full scope of general surgery.

Dr. Flint recruited Dr. Jaffe to come to Tulane from SUNY in 1992. Drs. Flint and Jaffe had shared a long friendship in New York, but their relationship actually started when Flint was interviewing for his surgical internship at Barnes Hospital—a young Dr. Jaffe was assigned to give him a tour, and they remained close friends after. While Dr. Jaffe was a general surgeon, he often worked with the specialists in their fields as well. Dr. Jaffe was one of the first surgeons to perform living-related

---

174 Interview with Lewis Flint, July 23, 2010.
175 Interview with Norman McSwain, November 16, 2012.

donor small bowel transplants.[176] In a time of vast changes in trauma resuscitation, he also worked with Dr. McSwain and the Charity faculty to define new recommendations. In one such anecdote, Drs. McSwain and Jaffe were rounding on patients in Charity on the Saturday before Mardi Gras. One particular patient was not doing well, and they ordered a battery of tests and scans. Unfortunately, Drs. McSwain and Jaffe had to leave to ride in the Endymion parade. With the parade route being so loud, they would never be able to hear the test results over the phone. The residents decided to find cardboard posters and write the results in large print so that they could be read from McSwain and Jaffe's parade float. After seeing the results on the parade route, they called orders in by phone to the residents, and the patient did marvelously.[177]

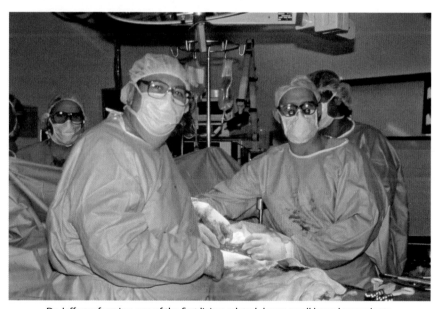

Dr. Jaffe performing one of the first living-related donor small bowel transplants.

176 Interview with Bernard Jaffe, November 14, 2012.
177 Interview with Bernard Jaffe, November 14, 2012.

The Department of Surgery developed its multiorgan transplant program under the guidance of Dr. Douglas Slakey, who was director of the Tulane Center for Abdominal Transplantation from 1998 until 2006. Dr. Slakey and Tulane have been pioneers in the area of laparoscopic living donor nephrectomy. In 1997, Dr. Slakey performed the first laparoscopic living donor nephrectomy for renal transplant in the southeastern United States at Tulane University Hospital and Clinic.

Along with Dr. Slakey, Dr. Flint also recruited Dr. Stephen Cheng and Dr. Frederick Regenstein. After their arrivals, Drs. Slakey and Cheng established the certification for liver transplants at Tulane, which had been problematic for the department in the past. This time around, it was acquired in twenty-four months, the minimum amount of time and, still to this day, the fastest any program has acquired certification. In 1999 Drs. Slakey and Cheng began a pediatric living donor liver transplant program, which had 100 percent one-year survival. With the multiorgan program, Tulane's leadership has been seen in the area of liver, pancreas, and kidney transplants, and the program experienced rapid growth from 60 transplants in 1997 to 216 transplants in 2004.[178] Today, Dr. Jennifer McGee is conducting research into outcome disparities by race and gender in kidney transplantation, which will assist future surgeons in better understanding these important factors in transplantation success rates.

In 1999, Dr. Flint left Tulane to become the director of trauma and surgical critical care at the University of South Florida. Today, he is the editor of the American College of Surgeons *Selected Readings in General Surgery*.

---

178 Organ Procurement and Transplant Network, US Department of Health and Human Services, UNOS/OPTN data, http://optn.transplant.hrsa.gov, (accessed December 28, 2012).

Robert L. Hewitt, 2000–2006

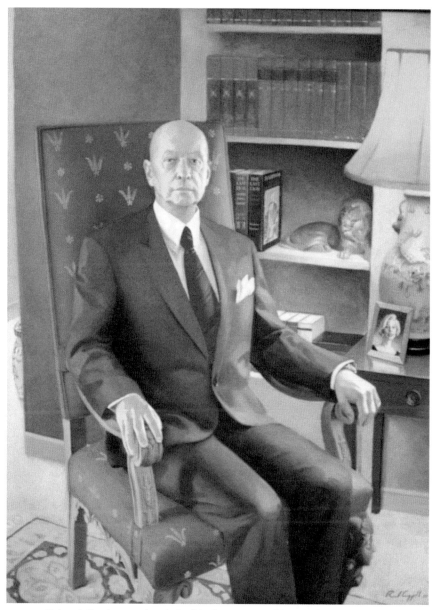

Robert L. Hewitt served as chair of the Department of Surgery from 2000–2006.

Dr. Robert L. Hewitt, who had received his MD from Tulane in 1959 and completed his residency at the university before joining the staff in 1968, was selected as the next chair of the Department of Surgery in 2000. In 1970, Dr. Hewitt became the chief of the cardiac surgery division within the department until 1976, when he entered private practice. He maintained his affiliation with Tulane and returned to the faculty in 1994. Dr. Hewitt had a style that was completely different from Dr. Flint. While Flint was highly academic, introverted, and very opinionated on how the department should be run, Hewitt was just the opposite. Hewitt was very laid back, was friendly, had many connections with surgeons and others in the community from his time in private practice, and had a laissez-faire attitude while running the department.[179]

Upon assuming the chair of surgery, Tulane charged Dr. Hewitt with rebuilding and reorganizing the department.[180] Support from the medical school, the university, and Tulane University Hospital and the recruitment of faculty in a number of specialty areas made such progress possible. The department established a section of surgical oncology with special attention on breast disease and placed an emphasis on cardiac transplantation and cardiac surgery, for both acquired and congenital conditions.

In 1993, the Tulane Cancer Center had been established, which was followed by the Tulane Cancer Center Comprehensive Clinic, a state-of-the-art multidisciplinary treatment facility within Tulane University Hospital. Tulane also partnered with the LSU Health Sciences Center to form the Louisiana Cancer Research Consortium in 2002. Surgery department faculty were active in the clinical and research programs of the cancer center. For example, the work of Dr. Bernard Jaffe in recognizing the usefulness of calcium channel blockers in combating the physiological effects of the hormones involved in carcinoid

179 Interview with Bernard Jaffe, November 14, 2012.
180 Interview with Ronald Nichols, November 13, 2012.

syndrome has changed the way carcinoid patients are cared for. The use of those calcium blockers in treating the symptoms of the syndrome has been met with great success.

Another area of general surgery where Tulane has established itself as a leader is minimally invasive, or laparoscopic, surgery. Dr. Robert Hewitt's tenure as departmental chair saw the enhancement of laparoscopic surgery with the establishment of a new surgical skills laboratory and the Minimally Invasive Surgical Center, which included teaching, research, and clinical programs. Today, the Tulane Center for Advanced Medical Simulation and Team Training, directed by Dr. James Korndorffer, offers enhanced training with Stryker High Definition Laparoscopic trainers. Success with these programs led to the acquisition of robotic surgery at Tulane University Hospital.

Dr. Hewitt was chair of the department during the devastation of New Orleans following Hurricanes Katrina and Rita. He retired in January 2006, after fifty years of association with the Tulane School of Medicine.

Douglas P. Slakey, 2006–

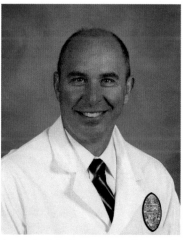

Douglas P. Slakey served as chair of the Department of Surgery from 2006 to the present.

Dr. Douglas Slakey assumed the leadership of the department following Dr. Hewitt's retirement. Having received his medical degree and general surgery residency from the Medical College of Wisconsin and transplantation fellowships from John Hopkins University and Oxford University, England, Dr. Slakey joined the Tulane School of Medicine as director of the Tulane Center for Abdominal Transplantation in 1997. Dr. Slakey is widely respected for his pioneering efforts in laparoscopic surgery. He was the first surgeon in the southeastern United States to perform laparoscopic living donor nephrectomy for renal transplantation and one of the first to perform major laparoscopic liver resections.[181]

With the uncertainty and problems with communication that immediately followed Hurricanes Katrina and Rita, a website for the transplantation section that had been established by Dr. Slakey and housed on a server in Alabama became a means of communication for surgery faculty, residents, referring physicians, and patients. With the medical school and Tulane Hospital closed following the storm, Tulane surgical faculty worked to establish satellite clinics along the Gulf Coast in Louisiana, Mississippi, and Florida.[182]

Following Hurricanes Katrina and Rita, the department restarted the transplantation program soon after Valentine's Day 2006, when a living donor surgery was done involving a husband-and-wife couple named the Harts. Since then, the program has continued its leadership role. In 2006, Tulane launched a national organ donor program called the Give Five–Save Lives initiative. The program was announced at the National Learning Congress on Organ Donation and Transplantation held at Tulane and serves to stimulate organ donations by helping businesses

---

181 Sarah Balyeat, "Douglas Slakey, MD, MPH, FACS: A Pioneer of Laparoscopic Living Donor Transplant Procedures," *Tulane Transplant Times* (Summer 2007), p. 2.
182 Interview with Douglas Slakey, August 20, 2010.

and organizations educate their employees about organ and tissue donation.[183]

The Tulane Department of Surgery has continued its recovery from the hurricanes of 2005 under Dr. Slakey's leadership. The Department of Surgery was left with seven full-time faculty following the exodus from the storms and the release of faculty during Tulane's post-Katrina renewal program. Thus, faculty retention and recruitment have been emphasized since 2006, with twenty-three new full-time faculty and additional clinical staff added to the department during Dr. Slakey's tenure.

During that time the department established the first academic endocrine surgery section in the region and continued to focus on minimally invasive surgery. Growth in the area of laparoscopic surgery led to the development of robotic surgery at Tulane University Hospital. Dr. Emad Kandil, chief of endocrine surgery, has advanced robotic endocrine surgery. Dr. Kandil's technique of performing thyroidectomies by using a robotic system and incisions under the arm rather than the traditional larger incision in the neck has garnered national and international attention.

Dr. Juan C. Duchesne was also attracted after Katrina; Duchesne, along with Drs. Norman McSwain and Peter Meade, is conducting important research in the areas of damage control resuscitation and damage control surgery. These new approaches to resuscitating and caring for trauma patients focus on the initial steps of controlling hemorrhage, preventing contaminants, and safeguarding from further injury until a patient can be better resuscitated. The patient later undergoes a definitive surgical procedure when he or she is better able to withstand the rigors of surgery.

During the mid-1990s, Charity Hospital was designated a Level 1 trauma center due, in many ways, to the service of faculty from the Tulane Department of Surgery. Although it held

---

183 Ted Griggs, "Tulane Launches Nat'l Organ Donor Program." *Acadiana Medical News* (December 2006), p. 1–2.

a long-standing position of service within the department, the section of trauma and critical care was not formally established until 2009, having been for many years connected to general surgery instruction and care.

In 2006, the Tulane Department of Surgery recognized the need to reorganize its residency program following the decision by the Residency Review Committee of the Accreditation Council for Graduate Medical Education (ACGME) that population levels in the New Orleans area did not warrant three programs and that Tulane's residency program should be closed. Rather than protest this decision, the department decided to voluntarily close its residency program and submit an application for a new program. Such a decision had only been successfully accomplished by a medical institution twice before, but in June 2007, the RRC approved the application, thanks to leadership provided by department chair Douglas Slakey and Jim Korndorffer. Following its temporary one-year approval, the RRC reaccredited the residency program in early 2009. During the 2009 site visit, the department received no citations and was placed on a five-year accreditation cycle.[184]

The residency curriculum currently encompasses clinical rotations in seven area hospitals: Tulane Medical Center, Tulane Lakeside Hospital, MCLNO University Hospital, Children's Hospital, East Jefferson General Hospital, Touro Medical Center, and West Jefferson General Hospital. These institutions provide residents with diverse clinical settings, surgical cases, and patient populations. Structured on six competencies established by the ACGME, Tulane's residency program provides training and evaluation of residents in the areas of patient care, medical knowledge, practice-based learning and improvement, interpersonal and communication skills, professionalism, and systems-based practice. Clinical rotations, ranging from one to four months, cover all areas of general surgery and are intended to provide a graduated level of responsibility

---

184 Interview with Douglas Slakey, August 20, 2010.

and training during the five-year program. The Tulane surgery residency has recovered from the challenges faced after Hurricane Katrina and has regained its reputation as a premier surgical training program. As an example, in 2012, the program had 974 applicants, representing 111 US medical schools, for four categorical positions.

Apart from faculty recruitment, another focus of the department in the post-Katrina era has been the development of strategies to build patient and clinical volume and to strengthen the surgery curriculum for residents and medical students. One approach has been to look for areas of cooperation with other health care providers in the greater New Orleans region. Under the guidance of Dr. Slakey and Dr. Patrick O'Leary, chairman of LSU's department of surgery, the trauma service at University Hospital merged into one service with students, residents, and faculty from both institutions working together. Previously, trauma service provided by Tulane and LSU at the hospital had been strictly divided. The same merger arrangement has been implemented for pediatric surgery, plastic surgery, and transplant surgery. It is hoped that this model of service will serve to reduce competition and redundancy between the two schools, provide a higher quality of service to patients, and eliminate some of the politics that Dr. Ochsner and other chairs had protested.

The Tulane Department of Surgery has had a long and storied history, filled with tribulations and triumphs. From pioneering major advances in the field of surgery to having the first department chairs dueling outside the grounds of Charity Hospital, from cultivating some of the greatest surgical innovators in history to massive destruction from Hurricane Katrina, Tulane has not only stood the trials of time, but has flourished with each newly encountered challenge.

Historical Timeline

1736
The first Charity Hospital opened in a house at Chartres and Bienville Streets on May 10.

1830
Future professor of surgery and dean Dr. Charles A. Luzenberg is the second Louisiana physician to perform a cesarean section.

1833
Dr. Warren Stone discovered the benefit of cold water, used internally and externally, for cholera patients while treating patients at Charity Hospital.

1834
"The First Circular or Prospectus of the Medical College of Louisiana" appeared in *L'Abeille* (The Bee) on September 29.

Dr. Luzenberg performed the first successful ligation of the common iliac artery for aneurysm performed at Charity Hospital

1835
Dr. Thomas Hunt delivered the first lecture of the Medical College of Louisiana in January.

Dr. Luzenberg became dean of the medical college.

1837
Following the resignation of Dr. Luzenberg, Dr. Stone was elected as professor and chair of surgery. He served in that position until April 1872.

1838
In April, an article entitled "Sight Given to the Born Blind" appeared in the *True American* and detailed an operation performed by Dr. Luzenberg on the eyes of a female Seminole patient. Controversy followed, and an inquiry was made into the publication of the article.

1844
The first permanent home of the medical college was built at the corner of Philippa and Common Streets.

1847
An act incorporated the medical college as the medical department of the University of Louisiana.

Dr. Stone performed the first successful amputation of the thigh under Letheon, or sulphuric ether, in Louisiana in February

1859
Dr. Stone was the first to apply a silver ligature to an artery.

1863 November–1965 November
The University of Louisiana was closed due to the Civil War.

1865
Dr. T. G. Richardson became the dean of the medical school.

1872
Dr. Richardson succeeded Warren Stone as professor of surgery.

1877
Dr. Richardson became the first doctor from Louisiana to serve as president of the American Medical Association.

1884
Legislative Act No. 42 created the Tulane University of Louisiana.

1886
The first premedical course was established at Tulane.

1888
Dr. Rudolph Matas performed the first operation of endoan-eurysmorrhaphy in a patient with traumatic aneurysm of the brachial artery.

1889
Dr. Samuel Logan was elected to chair of surgery, serving until 1892.

1892
Dr. Albert B. Miles succeeded Samuel Logan as chair of surgery for a year prior to his death from hemorrhagic typhoid fever in 1894.

1893
Following the death of T. G. Richardson, his wife, Ida, made a memorial gift of nearly one hundred and fifty thousand dollars to Tulane, which included a new building on Canal Street.

1894
Dr. Matas became chairman of surgery, serving until 1927.

1895
The A. B. Miles Surgical Amphitheatre at Charity Hospital was completed.

1902
Alexander Charles Hutchinson, a transportation executive and patient of Rudolph Matas, left his estate, valued at seven hundred and fifty thousand dollars, to the medical department.

1906
The New Orleans Polyclinic became the postgraduate medical department at Tulane University.

1916
The Tulane Unit, Base Hospital No. 24, was established. Staffed by professors and students from Tulane, the hospital served with distinction in France during World War I.

1927
Dr. Alton Ochsner succeeded Rudolph Matas as chair of the Department of Surgery, serving until 1956.

1930
The School of Medicine moved from the Hutchinson Building on Canal Street to the Hutchinson Memorial Building on Tulane Avenue.

A personal letter written by Dr. Ochsner describing the political nature of Charity Hospital was presented to Governor Huey P. Long and the hospital board, which resulted in the termination of Ochsner's appointment to the hospital's visiting staff.

1932
Tulane School of Medicine student and future Tulane surgeon Michael DeBakey invented the "roller pump," which became an essential component of the heart-lung machine that permitted open-heart surgery.

1934
Neal Owens became the first instructor of plastic surgery at Tulane University.

1936
On April 15, Dr. Ochsner performed the first pneumonectomy in the Deep South as a means of dealing with a malignant bronchial lesion.

Dr. Ochsner observed nine cases of carcinoma of the lung in a six-month period at Charity Hospital. His investigations and the determination that all the patients were heavy smokers led to Ochsner's early belief in the link between smoking and lung cancer.

1941
Dr. Ochsner, along with four colleagues at Tulane, founded the Ochsner Clinic.

1949
Dr. Ochsner performed the first operative procedure shown on closed-circuit television in New Orleans during a visit by the International Society of Surgery.

1956
A January 2 article in *Time* featuring Dr. Ochsner described, in part, his "bullpen."

Dr. Oscar Creech accepted the chair of the Department of Surgery.

1957
Edward Krementz, Oscar Creech, and Robert Ryan developed the regional perfusion technique, which was found to be beneficial in cases of malignant melanoma, pelvic cancers, and soft tissue sarcomas.
1959
Dr. Creech and a team of doctors from Tulane performed Louisiana's first kidney transplant using a kidney donated by Ned LeBlanc to his twin brother, Abel.

1963
During his Ivy Day speech, Dr. Creech called for the establishment of a university hospital.

Dr. Keith Reemtsma begins his pioneering and controversial xenotransplantations of chimpanzee kidneys to humans.

1967
Dr. Creech accepted the position of dean of the medical school in July and served until his death in December of that year.

Dr. Edward Krementz served as acting chairman of the Department of Surgery until Theodore Drapanas assumed the position on September 1, 1968.

1972
Dr. John C. McDonald and Dr. Theodore Drapanas performed the first liver transplant in Louisiana.

1975
Dr. Drapanas was killed in a plane crash. Dr. Robert Frank Ryan served as acting chairman during the search for Dr. Drapanas's replacement.

1976
The dedication of the Tulane Medical Center took place on September 23.

1977
Dr. Watts R. Webb joined the Tulane faculty as chairman of the department on May 1, serving until 1989.

1979
The first life-saving living donor pediatric kidney transplantation was performed at Tulane University Hospital for Children

on May 8. The pediatric renal transplantation program would go on to perform over 260 pediatric kidney transplants at the hospital.

1989
Dr. Lewis Flint became the chair of the department, serving until 1999.

2000
Dr. Robert Hewitt became the chair of the department, serving until 2006.

2005
Hurricanes Katrina and Rita devastated New Orleans, forcing the temporary closure of University Hospital and the Tulane School of Medicine.

2006
Dr. Douglas Slakey became the chair of the department, following Dr. Hewitt's retirement.

2006–2007
The Department of Surgery residency program was reorganized.

2009
The residency program was placed on a five-year accreditation cycle.

Tulane University Department of Surgery
Department Chairmen

Charles Aloysius Luzenberg, 1835–1837

Warren Stone, 1837–1872

Tobias Gibson   Richardson, 1872–1889

Samuel Logan, 1889–1893

Albert Baldwin Miles, 1893–1894

Rudolph Matas, 1895–1927

Edward William Alton Ochsner, 1927–1956

Oscar Creech Jr., 1956–1967

Edward Thomas Krementz, 1967–1968 (Acting)

Theodore Drapanas, 1968–1975

Robert Frank Ryan, 1975–1977 (Acting)

Watts Webb, 1977–1989

Lewis M. Flint, 1989–1999

Robert L. Hewitt, 2000–2006

Douglas P. Slakey, 2006–

Tulane University surgeons with roles in the American College of Surgeons

American College of Surgeons—Founders

Carroll W Allen
S.M.D. Clark
Marcus Feingold
Herman B Gessner
Ernest S Lewis
E. Denegre Martin
Rudolph Matas
Jeff Miller
Frederick Wm. Parham

American College of Surgeons—Presidents

Rudolph Matas, 1926
C. Jeff Miller, 1931
Alton Ochsner, 1951

American College of Surgeons—Officers

Rudolph Matas, 1913–1920, 1924–1925
C. Jeff Miller, 1930

American College of Surgeons—Advisory Council

Rudolph Matas, 1940–1956
Alton Ochsner, 1954–1980

American College of Surgeons—Board of Regents

Frederick W. Parham, 1922–1926
Jeff Miller, 1927–1936

Alton Ochsner, 1936–1952
Conrad G. Collins, 1962–1967

American College of Surgeons—Board of Governors

Charles Landfried, 1914–1915
Earnest S. Lewis, 1914–1915
Denegre Martin, 1914–1915
Rudolph Matas, 1914–1915
C. Jeff Miller, 1914–1928
Frederick W. Parham, 1914–1925
Robert C. Lynch, 1930–1932
Alton Ochsner, 1931–1936
Hilliard E. Miller, 1936–1945
Thomas B. Sellers, 1936–1953
I. Mims Gage, 1947–1954
Guy A. Caldwell, 1952–1954
Woodard Beacham, 1956–1963
Ambrose Storck, 1959–1961
Francis E. LeJeune, 1961–1963
Oscar Creech, Jr., 1962–1964
Harry D. Morris, 1962–1964
Joseph J. Noya, 1977–1982
Elmo J. Cerise, 1982–1986
Lewis M. Flint, 1993–1998
Robert H. Miller, 1997–1999

Made in United States
Orlando, FL
17 November 2021

10499250R00071